Erika Harvey was editor of *Here's Health* and *Parents* and now works as a freelance writer for various other health and childcare magazines, including *Pregnancy & Birth* and *Mother & Baby*. She is a member of the Guild of Health Writers.

YOUR CHILD SERIES

A series of books containing easy-to-follow, practical advice for the parents of children with a variety of illnesses or conditions.

Each book provides a clear overview of the situation, explaining essential information about the illness or condition and outlining the practical steps parents can take to help understand, support and care for their child, the rest of the family as well as themselves. Guiding parents through the conventional, the complementary and the alternative approaches available, these books cater for children of all ages, ranging from babies to teenagers, and enable the whole family to move forward in a positive way.

Other Books in the Series:

Your Child: Bullying by Jenny Alexander
Your Child: Diabetes by Catherine Steven
Your Child: Eczema by Maggie Jones

YOUR CHILD

Asthma
Practical and Easy-to-Follow Advice

Erika Harvey

ELEMENT

Shaftesbury, Dorset • Boston, Massachusetts
Melbourne, Victoria

© Element Books Limited 1998
Text © Erika Harvey 1998

First published in Great Britain in 1998 by
Element Books Limited
Shaftesbury, Dorset SP7 8BP

Published in the USA in 1998 by
Element Books, Inc.
160 North Washington Street
Boston, MA 02114

Published in Australia in 1998 by
Element Books and distributed
by Penguin Books Australia Ltd
487 Maroondah Highway, Ringwood,
Victoria 3134

Design by Roger Lightfoot
Typeset by Footnote Graphics, Warminster, Wilts
Printed and bound in Great Britain by
Creative Print and Design Wales, Ebbw Vale

British Library Cataloguing in Publication
data available

Library of Congress Cataloging in Publication
data available

ISBN 1 86204 207 1

£3

Contents

Introduction   vii

1   What is Asthma?   1
2   Helping Your Child   20
3   The Emotional Aspects of Asthma   38
4   Conventional Treatments   55
5   Complementary Approaches   71
6   As They Grow   88

Further Reading   110
Useful Addresses   111

Introduction

'Nicola started off just coughing and wheezing. A cold, we thought. During the night, it got steadily worse and then, very quickly – in minutes – she was choking for breath. She couldn't talk. She was terribly frightened about what was happening and I couldn't calm her because I was panicking, too. The journey to casualty was the longest in my life, listening to her gasping attempts to get air. I thought she was going to die in my arms. At the hospital, they knew immediately what it was and what to do. I couldn't believe it when they told me it was an asthma attack. Nicola didn't suffer from asthma.'

This is how one mother describes her daughter's first asthma attack. It happened three years ago when Nicola was seven years old, but her mother still remembers every terrifying detail and the anguished gamut of feelings – the fear, disbelief, desperation and guilt that it might have been something she did or did not do which triggered the attack.

Talking to parents of asthmatic children, one finds that these feelings are common, and none of them forgets the terror of that first attack – particularly if they have had no previous brush with the condition. An asthma attack is a frightening experience for everyone concerned, whether it is the first, second or fiftieth time it has occurred. For the person suffering the attack, it is a gasping, painful struggle to get air into your lungs. Parents of a child going through an asthma attack feel like terrified bystanders, desperate to do something, aware that the need to breathe is paramount but feeling unable to help their child.

It is not always like this; most children suffer from asthma mildly, which means that they only occasionally have symptoms, usually following exposure to a trigger like cold air or exercise. Or they may have low-level symptoms – a cough or wheezing – most of the time, but these tend not to reach the critical level of an actual attack. Asthma is a very changeable beast. It varies in severity from individual to individual and from attack to attack and is brought on by different triggers in different people and at different times. It can develop at any time in susceptible children and they can also grow out of it, mostly as they go into adolescence, although they will always have an 'asthma tendency' and it may recur later in life.

If your child has asthma, then he or she is not alone. More and more parents are becoming acquainted with the condition, as it is on the rise worldwide: the number of children diagnosed as asthmatic has doubled since 1970. Figures gathered by the International Study of Asthma and Allergy in Children (ISAAC) show that the USA, Australia, New Zealand and the UK have the highest rates in the world for older children with asthma (the study looked at 14-year-olds), while Canada, Japan, Latin America and Australia have the highest rates for younger children. Australia has the overall highest rate of childhood asthma, with estimates putting it at around 30 per cent. It is estimated to affect around 1.5 million children – one in 7 – in the UK alone.

Epidemiologists and other experts have a wealth of statistical evidence to show that asthma is a growing, worldwide problem; what they do not yet have is a clear reason why it has leapt to pandemic proportions over the last 20 years or so. Part of the reason may be that parents are now more aware of asthma and seek help and treatment earlier; doctors themselves are also diagnosing it more frequently than in the past. In addition, it is possible that other respiratory disorders have now been recategorized as asthma. Beyond this, there is, we know, a definite and long-established genetic susceptibility involved in the development of asthma. If one parent is asthmatic, there is at least a 25 per cent likelihood that a child will develop it; if both parents suffer from asthma, then the chances rise to 50 per cent.

Asthma is also an allergy-related condition and a family history of other atopic problems like eczema, rhinitis or hay fever puts your child at an increased risk of developing asthma – and vice versa: around 40 per cent of children with asthma also have eczema. It seems hard that children already suffering a chronic respiratory condition should also have to put up with the discomfort of eczema, but it fits in with the pattern of oversensitivity that some children experience.

Bearing in mind both the genetic link and the current global rise, it looks as though more children will develop the condition as this generation grows up, become parents in their turn and pass their susceptibility on to their children. Asthma is rapidly becoming a condition which will touch the majority of us at some point in our lives, whether it is as parents or as grandparents.

Breathing is our most basic instinct: breath is life. Asthma stops us taking this instinctual function for granted – it robs us of air and so has the potential to rob us of life, too. Although death from asthma is rare in childhood, it is still fatal for an estimated 30 children in a year. If you live with the nagging worry that some harmless action, exertion or outing may trigger an attack, it is easy to wrap a child in cotton wool and change her life to accommodate the asthma, even though what parents want – and want to work towards – is for their child to live a normal life.

The good news is that, for most children with asthma, it is possible to live a normal life, to do all the things their friends do and feel confident that it will not bring on either symptoms or an attack. This is in a large part thanks to the fact that, although the conventional treatments currently available cannot cure the condition, they can control it very effectively. Complementary therapies also have an important role to play, in boosting the immune system and stimulating the body's own natural powers to fight the illness. In addition, as we learn more about what triggers asthma, we can root out the culprits and make changes to a child's environment, diet and lifestyle which minimize the chances of an attack. In this way, parents can make a big difference to their child's life.

How *you* can make a difference to your child's asthma is the main focus of this book. Although it covers all the important medical information, like what happens in the body to cause asthma symptoms, the triggers and the treatments, it also offers you practical ways to alleviate symptoms and feel in control of the condition. In addition, you will find a comprehensive guide to complementary therapies which can help the condition, even in some cases enabling your child to leave off medication altogether once the complementary treatment shows results.

The book also covers the emotional side of having a child with asthma in the family: what problems he is likely to come across and how you can beat them in a positive, united way; the effects of stress and how to put it into perspective; and, of course, advice on letting your child become more independent as he grows older.

Asthma is certainly not a life sentence. Given all the options, your child can enjoy life to the full. All you need is a willingness to make changes in your life to help her, an open mind towards treatment, both conventional and complementary, a positive attitude, and a rock-solid determination that asthma will not rule the roost in your home!

Note. To avoid clumsy constructions, the pronouns 'he' and 'she' are used in alternate chapters when the sex of the child is indeterminate, and should be taken to indicate both genders.

Chapter One

What is Asthma?

Asthma is basically an inflammatory condition of the lungs, where the airways swell up, the muscles around them contract and air is prevented from getting through to those parts of the lungs responsible for feeding oxygen into the bloodstream. The severity of the problem depends on how closed the airways become. A mild attack may cause coughing and some breathlessness; in a very severe attack, levels of oxygen in the blood can become so low that a child loses consciousness, although this is very rare. This inflammation develops because the body is hypersensitive to something in the environment which would normally have no effect. It could be due to an allergic reaction to a substance known as an allergen or an oversensitive response to environmental conditions like air pollution or cold air, or it could be brought on by exercise or an infection like a cold.

This sensitized reaction to a trigger causes three distinct symptoms to develop:

- The lining of the airways becomes inflamed and swollen, so they are narrower than normal.
- The muscles around the airways go into spasm (known as bronchospasm or bronchoconstriction), which narrows the airways even more.
- Quantities of thick, sticky mucus is produced in response to the inflammation and this effectively plugs up the airways.

The Inside Story

Your lungs, which sit on either side of your chest protected by your ribcage, carry out the job of supplying the body with oxygen and expelling carbon dioxide. Air is drawn into the lungs with the help of the ribs and diaphragm, a band of muscle which lies under the lungs. Air comes down the trachea (windpipe) and enters the two main airways (bronchi) into each lung. These airways branch into smaller and smaller airways until they reach the alveoli, or air spaces, where oxygen is passed into the bloodstream. Carbon dioxide, meanwhile, passes out in the opposite direction as we exhale. In asthma, it is the airways which become inflamed and constricted, so oxygen does not get through to the alveoli.

ESTABLISHED TRIGGERS

The root cause of this bronchial chain reaction – that is, what sets up the sensitivity in the first place – has still not been clearly established, although science has got as far as tracking down a possible asthma gene. In the future, this could help in the development of a cure while providing a way to test people to find out if they are at risk.

What is becoming clearer is the extent to which the immune system is involved in the development of asthma. It appears to misfire in some way; it mistakes a normally harmless substance (like pollens or pet dander) for something harmful and develops antibodies – the body's defence against dangerous intruders like bacteria and viruses – against it. It is this malfunction in our defensive mechanism which lies at the root of all allergy-related conditions and which causes the symptoms of asthma to develop.

The 20th century does seem to be putting the immune system under pressure: generally, there has been a rise in allergy-related conditions, from asthma, eczema and hay fever to inflammatory bowel disorders and coeliac disease (where a person is intolerant of the gluten in wheat). In addition, although the genetic link is strong, an increasing number of people are developing an allergy-related condition when there is no family history of allergies. For this reason, researchers are now looking beyond genetics to pinpoint possible triggers in our environment.

In what follows, you will find the well-established triggers for asthma, while the next section looks at some new ones, for which evidence is still accumulating but which appear to show a link. If you are going to put into practice the steps covered in more detail in chapter 2, then you will need to think closely about what triggers your child is susceptible to, to narrow down the field a little. The chances are that he will not just react to a solitary trigger but to a combination. However, the main culprits are viral infections like colds (particularly in young children), pollens, pets and microscopic pests called house-dust mites.

Colds and other infections

In young children especially, the first asthma attack can follow a viral infection like a cold, and from then on, colds will act as triggers to future attacks. The obvious connection here is that the respiratory tract is usually implicated in a cold (sore throat, swollen glands, inflamed airways). Colds in young children also often lead to a bronchial infection, and the build-up of mucus in the area adds to the problem. When a cold becomes a perennial trigger for an asthma attack, it could be that the original viral infection left behind a weakness in the respiratory area which makes it more susceptible to subsequent colds and also other allergens.

More controversially, there is some research to indicate that, in some instances, asthma may be caused by traces of a virus taking up residence in the respiratory area. Research from the University Medical Centre in Ljubljana, Slovenia, focused on the adeno-virus bug, which causes an acute bronchial infection, as this has been implicated in the development of asthma. Researchers found that of 34 children who had an acute adenoviral infection and went on to develop asthma, 31 still had traces of the adenovirus bug in their lungs; they found no sign of the bug in children who did not develop asthma after the infection.

House-dust mites

These tiny bugs are among the most common triggers for asthma – thought to affect around 75 per cent of asthma sufferers – and unfortunately one of the hardest to avoid, since they inhabit every home and take up residence in their millions. The substance which causes the reaction – the allergen – is not the house-dust mite itself, but is found in its droppings. The mites live off us – off the microscopic skin flakes which we constantly shed – and in any occupied home this supplies them with a never-ending source of food. They colonize those places where we spend a lot of time: in mattresses, bedding, cushions, carpets, upholstery, cuddly toys, even clothes.

Animal dander (fur, hair, etc)

Because animals are thought to affect up to 40 per cent of children with asthma, any family with an asthmatic child should think long and hard before introducing a pet into the house.

Case Study
Pippa's son Matty, aged five, started to wheeze every time they paid an extended visit to his grandparents. Finally, he suffered a severe asthma attack which kept him overnight in hospital. Pippa is certain that Matty's asthma symptoms are linked to his grandparents' pets – two dogs and three cats – as he only develops asthma when he visits them. 'It's a pity because, even though my mother keeps the place spotless, we can't go there to stay. It only takes a few hours for Matty to start wheezing and calling for his inhaler,' says Pippa.

Pollen

Like people who suffer hay fever, asthmatic children are often very sensitive to pollens and a high pollen count can either trigger an attack or make the symptoms of asthma much worse. Pollens of one kind or another are in the air from February right through to October, so summer can be a miserable time for hay fever and asthma sufferers alike (and many people with asthma also have to put up with hay fever symptoms).

In spring and early summer, wind-pollinated plants release their pollens into the air. The most common pollen allergens are found in grasses, weeds like mugwort and ragweed, and rapeseed. In autumn, mould spores are thrown into the air by rotting vegetation and these, too, are common allergens for many people, so it is not until the colder winter weather sets in that some people find relief from hay fever and asthma symptoms.

Passive smoking

Cigarette smoke is proving to be a long-underestimated trigger for asthma. Recent studies have shown clear links between the development of asthma in children and mothers who smoked while pregnant, and children in households where there is a smoker are more likely to develop asthma. Researchers from the National Institute of Public Health in Oslo, Norway, investigated 3,754 infants born in 1992–93 and followed their progress for two years. They found that exposure to tobacco smoke increased a baby's risk of developing respiratory problems by about 50 per cent. For children with asthma, smoky environments have been shown to make the condition worse and lengthen recovery times after an attack, with a higher need for medication and more persistent symptoms. If your child has asthma, it really is vital that neither parent smokes and that he is kept away as much as possible from smoky environments.

Exercise

Many asthmatic children suffer what is known as exercise-induced asthma, which means that the condition tends to come on or be exacerbated by exercise, either during the activity itself or directly afterwards. It affects about 90 per cent of people with chronic asthma and 40 per cent of those with mild symptoms.

People who suffer exercise-induced asthma find that five to ten minutes into the exercise they start coughing and wheezing and experience tightness in the chest.

Case Study
'Being breathless and wheezing after running around was one of the things that made us suspect Paul had asthma,' says his mother Laura. 'He would try to keep up with his brothers, but he regularly had to give up and come back. The times he spent sitting with me at the playpark, huffing and wheezing, while Don and Alex went wild.'

The dilemma for most parents is that asthmatic children need exercise: it helps strengthen their bodies, keeps them fit, generates a sense of well-being and can counteract the effects of any stress in their lives. The fitter and stronger a child is, the fewer symptoms will occur. Children's bodies also produce growth hormone when they exercise, which is of particular importance to those with asthma because their growth may lag behind that of other children their age. Nowadays, however, most asthmatics can control exercise-induced symptoms with medication, so there is no reason for your child not to exercise.

Weather conditions

Very cold air, or moving from cold to warm air, exacerbates many people's asthma, probably because extremes of temperature irritate their oversensitive airways. Thunderstorms sometimes also lead to an increase in symptoms. A 1994 analysis of calls to a doctors' out-of-hours service on one storm-racked night across south-eastern and eastern England, reported in the British *Journal of Epidemiology and Community Health*, showed that one in four calls to the service concerned asthma. No one is sure why some thunderstorms have this effect; it could be changes in air pressure or humidity during a storm, complicating conditions (eg hot, dry weather before the storm), or simply the fact that the turbulence throws more allergens and pollens into the air.

Cockroaches

In the USA, scientists have put the rise in childhood asthma down to a cockroach epidemic sweeping the country. In a study of 1500 children in seven US cities, researchers found these nasty little bugs caused more allergic asthma reactions in inner-city children than house-dust mites or cats.

Stress and other emotions

Stress is another common trigger for asthma, and children can be just as stressed as adults, although the reasons are obviously different. For adults, most stress can be put down to work; for children, it may be pressure of schoolwork, the changes of puberty, problems with their peers (fitting in, girl/boyfriends) and, of course, examinations. For younger children, stress points can be starting playschool or school, changing schools, the death of a pet, a new baby in the family, even going on holiday or visiting friends or family the child does not know well. Children can also become stressed with frustration at not being able to do some task or activity – riding a bicycle, doing a puzzle or learning to read, for example.

Stress has a very profound effect on the body's systems: digestion shuts down, blood pressure goes up, muscles tense, heart rate increases and breathing rate speeds up as more oxygen is brought into the body for energy. Stress puts the body into overdrive and it is hardly surprising that symptoms of asthma develop where there is a susceptibility.

Other emotions can also affect asthma – laughter, excitement, even sadness and depression. Researchers at the State University of New York in Buffalo, USA, looked at 24 asthmatic children aged 8–17 to see how different extremes of emotion – happiness and sadness – affected their condition. The test involved the children watching scenes from the film *ET The Extra-Terrestrial*. Researchers found that, although being happy had no effect on symptoms, sadness appeared to affect the children's heart rate and respiratory stability directly.

20TH-CENTURY TRIGGERS

So much for the more established triggers; but what else could account for the rapid rise in asthma cases which has occurred in the last half of this century? Is there some aspect of modern living which is increasing our susceptibility to it, as well as to the other allergy-related disorders? At the moment, the following have staked a claim as possible triggers and research continues to establish exactly what effect they are having on our allergic responses and immune system.

Modern housing

Asthma is associated with damp living conditions, with symptoms caused by mould spores in the air. This is a problem that is more likely to be faced by children in poorer inner-city areas, where housing may be of a low standard and in bad repair, with pollution levels adding to the problem.

At the other extreme, asthma may also be caused by the most comfortable, energy-efficient environments. These days our homes are virtually sealed units, protected by double glazing and insulation, and kept warm by central heating rather than open fires and hot-water bottles. The other side of the coin is that this means poor ventilation, stale air, an accumulation of dust and a build-up of often toxic household chemicals, from carbon monoxide and sulphur dioxide to formaldehyde from furnishings. If there is a smoker in the house, the situation worsens.

Experts believe that air in a home should be renewed roughly every 30 minutes; when we had open fireplaces and chimneys, air was renewed every few minutes; nowadays, in winter in a modern, centrally heated home, the air may only enjoy a complete change every ten hours.

A number of studies have linked central heating to asthma symptoms. A German study, reported in the *British Medical Journal*, found that children living in homes with central heating are twice as likely to have asthma as those living in non-centrally heated homes. The reason for this may be that warmer houses encourage house-dust mites, so that there is a greater concentration, although going from cold air to warm in winter may also play a part.

Gas stoves have also been associated with an increased risk of asthma; the reason is thought to be the nitrogen dioxide which they throw out.

Frequent house moves

A recent Scottish study of 1,801 children in Inverness and Aberdeen looking into factors which increase children's likelihood of developing asthma surprisingly found that frequent house moves were more of a risk factor than air pollution or pet ownership. The authors of the study put forward the theory that moving house a lot in a child's early years exposes them to a steady supply of new environmental allergens, which make them more susceptible to asthma.

Air pollution

Many studies have shown links between air pollution and asthma, and it seems that even moderate levels can have an effect. Our bodies are having to process a heavy burden of toxins from the air, which could be compromising our immunity as well as irritating our respiratory system; it is estimated, for instance, that we are exposed to 1,000 times more lead in the air than our prehistoric ancestors, owing to car exhaust fumes and heavy industrial pollutants. We are also beginning to have a major problem with low-level ozone in big cities. In some cities air quality is so poor that it is a danger to health, and citizens are advised not to come into the city for work or tourism. With a growing bank of evidence to show that air pollution is implicated in a major way with respiratory problems, doctors and scientists in both the UK and the USA are now calling for their respective governments to adopt stricter air quality standards to protect people with asthma.

Chemical residues

Air is not the only way that pollutants enter our bodies; they get into the system in the water we drink and the food we eat.

Concerns about the water supply mainly concern nitrates leaching into the water table from farmland, and industrial pollutants running into rivers and streams. The latest cause for concern is that oestrogens from the contraceptive pill and hormone replacement therapy are entering the water supply; it has been suggested that this may be a factor in the decline in male fertility.

Pesticides and chemical food additives have more or less become part of the food chain. In the UK, around 1 billion gallons of pesticides are sprayed onto crops every year and recent surveys have found residues of this chemical onslaught in 42 per cent of all fruit and vegetables and 31 per cent of milk. Pesticides and fungicides are highly toxic and, by taking in a minute amount every time we eat, you could say we are in the process of slowly poisoning ourselves.

In addition, other chemicals are used on fresh food to ripen it, or to keep it from going off while it is being transported to the shops, and chemicals are used to colour, preserve and flavour processed foods. These chemicals are associated with physiological reactions – for example, certain chemicals have been linked to hyperactivity and attention deficiency disorder in susceptible children. The relationship between asthma and chemical residues in food is less firmly established, but some additives like tartrazine (E102), carmoisine (E122) and sulphur dioxide (E220–E227) have been linked to its development.

Food allergies and intolerances

There is evidence that the symptoms of asthma – in fact, of any atopic condition – may sometimes be triggered by an allergy or intolerance towards a particular food or foods, although this is a hotly debated area. Some doctors and dietitians say it has little to do with asthma development; others place it high on the list of triggers. Accordingly, estimates of the number of people affected by food allergies and intolerances vary from 2 to 20 per cent. There does, however, appear to be a higher incidence of food intolerance in children under three, which – to look on the bright side – many manage to overcome as they grow up.

Allergy or intolerance – what is the difference?

An *allergy* occurs when something in the environment – inhaled, eaten, put on the skin or injected, as in an insect sting – causes the immune system to react dramatically, usually immediately and in a variety of ways: rashes, weals, swelling, a runny nose, sneezing, puffed eyes, nausea and vomiting, and rarely anaphylactic shock, a potentially fatal immune response when the body system literally shuts down. Because of the strength of an allergic reaction, you do not usually have to look far for the cause – for example, if you have an allergy to peanuts, the effect is usually immediate.

An intolerance or sensitivity is often harder to pin down because the symptoms may be delayed and less dramatic. Intolerances appear to be on the increase, possibly because of pollution, chemicals in foods (including natural chemicals like lactose and gluten), heavy-metal poisoning, stress, bottle feeding and poor diet, as well as hereditary factors which have sensitized the immune system so that it reacts in a low-level way to formerly harmless substances. Symptoms of an intolerance include weight problems, eczema, bowel problems, insomnia, fatigue, sore throat, hot and cold sweats, thrush, frequent colds and infections. The development of asthma has been linked with inhalant allergy (pollen, house-dust mites), food allergy and food intolerance.

Vaccinations

It is interesting that the rise in the incidence of asthma coincides with the growth in widespread inoculations, and there is some strong evidence to support a link. For example, according to the campaigning journal *What Doctors Don't Tell You*, the US government's Center for Disease Control and Prevention monitored the progress of 500,000 children across the USA, accumulating all the evidence they could find on the side-effects of the MMR (measles, mumps and rubella) and DTP (diphtheria, tetanus and whooping cough) injections. They identified 34 major side-effects, including asthma.

Another study, conducted at the Lung Research Laboratory in Oxford and Wakayama Medical Centre in Japan, discovered a link between the tuberculosis vaccination (BCG) and later development of asthma. Children who reacted only mildly to the vaccine were significantly more likely to develop asthma than those who had a strong response. A strong response to the vaccine indicates that the person has probably contracted a mild version of tuberculosis in the past. This led the researchers to conclude that having tuberculosis provided some protection against developing asthma.

What this seems to indicate is that infectious illnesses in childhood may protect us from asthma by making the immune system work more efficiently – almost like keeping it primed. Vaccinations protect us from these illnesses, but conversely may make us more susceptible to allergy-related disorders like asthma. This theory is borne out by studies in Britain and Italy (of 11,900 families and 1,659 students respectively), which each found that children with brothers and sisters suffered fewer allergy-related conditions, including asthma, than only children; the likeliest reason for this was that they were exposed to more childhood infections, which boosted their immunity.

This list of triggers is pretty exhaustive but even so, it does not cover everything. Something quite unexpected could start off your child's asthma or prompt an attack, from wood dust after a day in the woodwork class to inhaled chemicals.

Case Study
'I got a Saturday job in a hairdresser's, but something there – whether it was the chemicals from the perms or the hair – irritated my asthma and I had to give it up,' remembers 18-year-old Kirstie.

Different kinds of asthma
Your doctor may speak of chronic asthma or acute asthma. *Chronic asthma* refers to symptoms of asthma like wheezing, breathlessness or coughing, which are there almost constantly to a greater or lesser degree. *Acute asthma* is an actual asthma attack.

Asthma can also be categorized in terms of what triggers it, although this is not always helpful because asthma usually has a number of triggers which can cross categories – for example, a child who develops general symptoms due to an allergy to house-dust mites may become worse with exercise or a cold.

Extrinsic asthma, also called allergic or atopic asthma, is triggered by external allergens, that is to say substances in the child's environment which cause an allergic reaction, like pollens, animal dander, house-dust mites or a food allergy or intolerance. *Intrinsic asthma*, also called non-allergic or viral asthma, is not caused by an allergic reaction but by triggers like exercise, stress, cold air and – most commonly of all – an infection like a cold. *Occupational asthma* occurs as a result of a person's workplace or the type of work he does. Substances known to cause occupational asthma include wood dust, animals, many adhesives, spray paints and dyes. Occupational asthma is not something which affects children, except when the time comes to consider a career (for more on career choices, *see* chapter 6).

DIAGNOSING ASTHMA

Although doctors are becoming much better at spotting asthma, it is often parents themselves who suggest it as a cause of their child's problems. There are several reasons for this: first, doctors are busy, and secondly, your child may come to the surgery symptom-free, because the attack has come and gone or symptoms only come on at night. In young children (particularly under two years old), it can be difficult to differentiate asthma from an infection – around 30 per cent of children under five experience wheezing. For these reasons, it can take several visits and courses of antibiotics before a doctor realizes that the antibiotics are not working, the infection is fairly constant and something else must be to blame.

Case Study
'Chloe wheezed right from the start, coughing her little lungs out all through the night, unable to get any sleep,' says Val, mother of two-year-old Chloe. 'It seemed like, from the minute she was born, she had a cold that she couldn't shift. She was given antibiotics, which made no difference whatsoever, and apart from that my doctor didn't seem to know what else to do. Then, at about three months old, her breathing became very laboured and we took her straight to the hospital, where they put her on a nebulizer to help her to breathe. The doctor there said he thought it might be asthma. I felt terrible that it hadn't been spotted before.'

Parents are very important when it comes to diagnosing asthma in a child. You know your child best, so you are in a position to help your doctor by giving a definitive list of symptoms along with any suspected triggers and when the symptoms occur.

The common symptoms to look out for are:

- **Coughing.** A long-lasting cough, often worse at night or after exercise, is one of the strongest indicators of asthma.
- **Wheezing.** This is a whistling or hissing sound as your child breathes, and indicates that the airways are considerably narrowed.
- **Shortness of breath.** This occurs when normal breathing becomes more and more of a struggle through constricted and inflamed passages.
- **Chest tightness.** This is a common feeling as the airways narrow and mucus builds up in the area.

Your child might also experience: chest pains owing to the general constriction of the area, and there may be a lack of energy because not enough oxygen is getting into the bloodstream to create energy, so that all body systems slow down; or to the physical exertion of an asthma attack (the coughing, wheezing, and struggle to breath normally). Watch out, however, for severe lethargy and drowsiness if they are coupled with a worsening of symptoms and if medication does not appear to be working; this can indicate a very severe attack and you should call for emergency medical help immediately. Your child may not develop all these symptoms. In mild cases, he may only cough, mainly at night. Even wheezing – a symptom strongly associated with asthma for many years – is not always apparent if the airways are only slightly narrowed.

When to suspect asthma
You should suspect asthma if:
• your child cannot run around without coughing, wheezing or becoming breathless; in asthma, a child may become more breathless *after* he has stopped running around than when running
• the symptoms become worse at night; why this should be is not clear, but theories include a reaction to hormonal and chemical changes in the body that occur at night, reduced lung function and the simple fact that there can be a concentration of house-dust mites in the bedroom, in mattresses, duvets, pillows and cuddly toys
• your child has repeated episodes of coughing, wheezing and breathlessness through the year; regular episodes may indicate that the cause is asthma, as a cough will not clear up if it is caused by asthma and your child does not get appropriate treatment
• you can clearly associate the bouts of wheezing or breathlessness with a trigger, for example during exercise, after spending time in a smoky atmosphere, when he goes out in the cold, or during the pollen season.

If you suspect asthma, consult your doctor to confirm that your child has the condition so that you can start getting it under control. See a complementary practitioner at this point, too, so that he can start working on the symptoms and boosting your child's natural healing abilities as early as possible.

When a condition is not asthma
In young children, there are a number of infections and illnesses which can be confused with asthma.
• **Bronchiolitis.** This is a viral infection of the lungs to which babies are particularly prone. It causes wheezing and can take some time to clear up. It may trigger the initial development of asthma.

- **Bronchitis.** This is a viral infection of the lungs, usually caused by the same viruses as colds and flu. It causes symptoms very similar to asthma – coughing, wheezing, difficult breathing, and copious amounts of phlegm – but it should clear up within four weeks. Antibiotics are only prescribed if there is a secondary bacterial infection. It may also trigger the initial development of asthma.
- **Croup.** This is an infection of the larynx (voice box), often following a cold. Symptoms include breathlessness, a hoarse cry, a barking cough and wheezing.
- **Cystic fibrosis.** This is a hereditary condition affecting both the pancreas – which underproduces digestive enzymes so that nutrients from food are poorly absorbed – and the lungs, which overproduce mucus, leading to repeated chest infections. Cystic fibrosis cannot yet be cured (although the gene responsible for its development has been pinpointed), but the condition can be managed by supplying additional digestive enzymes and keeping the lungs as free of mucus as possible.
- **Enlarged adenoids.** These glands, which lie behind the ears, develop at around four to six years and can cause problems if they become infected, resulting in coughing, catarrh and middle-ear infections.
- **Whooping cough.** Although it is not as common now as it used to be, because of widespread vaccination, whooping cough is a serious infectious illness characterized by severe coughing with a 'whooping' sound at the end, breathlessness, a high temperature, nose-bleeds and vomiting. It lasts between two and ten weeks.

In addition to the above symptoms your doctor will also want to know:

- if there is anyone else in the family with either asthma or a related atopic condition like eczema, hay fever or food allergies
- if you can link symptoms to specific triggers like smoky atmospheres, the pollen season, pets, etc.

In an older child (over six years), your doctor may take a series of peak flow meter readings to see if there is much variation. Peak flow readings basically show how fast air is leaving the lungs when your child exhales (officially called his peak expiratory flow or PEF) and indicates how narrowed the airways are.

To measure PEF, your doctor will ask your child to blow into a small, hand-held meter. In a child with asthma, PEF will vary 15 per cent or more between readings. An improvement in PEF – as well as an improvement in general symptoms – once he is on anti-asthma medication will confirm that he has asthma. Once asthma is diagnosed, daily PEF readings – mornings and evenings – often become part of your child's management routine, as fluctuations in PEF (variations in readings of 15 per cent or more between two readings, with dips in the morning) are a good indicator that asthma is not being well controlled or an attack is imminent.

Your doctor will not try to take peak flow readings from children under six; it is simply too difficult to get an accurate reading and to get children to blow properly into the meter. He will rely on the other indicators of asthma outlined above to make a diagnosis.

▦ DRAWING UP A MANAGEMENT PLAN

Once your child has been diagnosed as asthmatic, you and your doctor or asthma nurse will draw up an asthma management plan together. These plans will vary according to the child and his asthma: the management plan for a child with mild asthma will be very different from one for a child who has severe symptoms which develop quickly. However, the basic plan should cover:

- how to recognize the signs of the condition becoming worse, and what steps to take
- how to step up the medication in the event of asthma symptoms worsening or your child having an attack
- when to call the doctor or take your child to the hospital
- what action to take in an emergency.

In older children, it will also include a record of peak flow readings and how to recognize whether or not they indicate a worsening of the condition. Your doctor or asthma nurse should give you special charts for plotting your child's PEF readings so you can see at a glance if they are starting to fluctuate or dip.

In the past, these plans have usually been drawn up informally, following a chat with the doctor. Now patients and doctors are encouraged to write down their plan, as it gives the patient or his parents something concrete to refer to at a time when he may be panicking and not thinking clearly.

Case Study

'I used to panic a lot,' admits Laura. 'But having a treatment plan for Paul has helped me to calm down when his symptoms start getting worse. Also, he can now give PEF readings, which he wasn't able to do when he was first diagnosed with asthma at three and a half. I've found this really helpful in spotting the signs that his asthma wasn't under control.'

Parents find it useful to have a step-by-step process to follow in the event of an attack and the plans help in deciding whether an asthma episode is an emergency or not. If your child does not have a management plan, talk to your doctor or asthma nurse about drawing one up.

GROWING OUT OF IT

The good news is that around one-third of children grow out of asthma in their teens, and for another third, the symptoms improve considerably or there are longer stretches between attacks. For the final third, however, asthma can dig its heels in and refuse to budge, although the symptoms may become milder. The younger a child develops asthma, the more likely he is to grow out of it (around two-thirds of children under five who develop asthma grow out of it). Moreover, children whose asthma is viral in origin rather than allergic tend to outgrow it, possibly because their airways are not under such constant attack as they are with allergic asthma and they have time to recover between infections. A child's resistance to infection also strengthens as he grows up.

How bad is it?

Asthma is usually divided into three levels of severity, but because it is such a changeable condition the severity may vary from one attack to another, or become milder or more severe over time. The constant factor in asthma is its chameleon nature. The levels are:

- **Mild asthma.** Occasional symptoms may include any one or more of the following: coughing, wheeziness, shortness of breath and tight chest. You can generally keep it under control with just a reliever drug, when symptoms come on; complementary treatment can help stop symptoms coming on.
- **Moderate asthma.** The condition is more chronic (symptoms are more constant) and it fluctuates, with quite severe flare-ups. There may be a number of triggers. Your doctor will probably advise both daily preventive drugs and relievers and a short course of steroid tablets when necessary.
- **Severe asthma.** The symptoms interfere with your child's life to a greater extent, with some severe flare-ups. Your doctor may advise higher-dose preventive medication, plus relievers. With both moderate and severe asthma, complementary therapies can help your child considerably.
- **Brittle asthma** is the most severe form of the condition. It involves a serious attack with no prior warning signs, but is, thankfully, rare.

For more on action during a severe asthma attack and signs of an emergency, *see* chapter 4.

Chapter Two

Helping Your Child

When your child is first diagnosed as having asthma, the first thing you think of as a parent is: how can I help her? The good news is that there is a lot you can do. First, you can help her to avoid the triggers which prompt her asthma symptoms. Secondly, you can ensure that her asthma is well controlled and her life as uninterrupted by the condition as possible. Thirdly, you can underpin her progress by taking her to see a complementary therapist. Fourthly, you can support her through the bad times, know when to let her take responsibility for her asthma, and keep an eye out for signs that she is not coping emotionally as well as usual.

This chapter is concerned with the practical steps you can take to cut down on your child's exposure to allergens like house-dust mites, pollens and pet dander as well as pinpointing possible food intolerances. Later chapters deal with the emotional side of having an asthmatic child in the family, and getting the treatment – both conventional and complementary – just right.

Before you rush off to put into practice all the suggestions which follow, however, first decide which ones will help in your child's particular case. Since most of the tips are to do with cutting down on allergens, make sure that your child's asthma is triggered by that particular allergen, otherwise you may be wasting your time. If you know she is affected by the allergen being discussed then the measures here are certainly worthwhile and may also have the knock-on effect of creating a friendlier, less reactionary environment for brothers and sisters who do not have asthma but who may also be susceptible to developing it.

Case Study
'I'd read an article which placed the blame for asthma on house-dust mites and it really struck a chord for me with Tamsin's asthma,' remembers Gaynor. 'So I blitzed the house. The first thing I did was put all her bedding – including the mattress – into special covers. I took the carpet out of her bedroom and put in lino, and got rid of all her fluffy toys, except her favourites. Her medication was not keeping up with her symptoms – she was wheezing and coughing in spite of being on a higher dose – and I was scared we would have to step up the steroids again, which I wanted to avoid. Thank goodness, the measures did seem to make a difference, particularly at night. I haven't really changed much in the rest of the house, although I vacuum every day and dust, and that seems to help, too. At least, I've noticed that if we stay away from home, her asthma gets worse and I can only think it's the changes I've made at home which keep her asthma at bay.'

Tracking down a trigger
- If you believe your child has allergic asthma, you could try a skin-prick test to isolate the allergen. This involves a tiny amount of the suspected allergens – or if none is specifically suspected, then the most common ones – being put under the skin. If a red weal or raised patch develops on the site, then your child has had a reaction and you have found a possible allergen.
- Alternatively, keep a symptom diary. List suspected allergens, activities, foods and so on, for example contact with animals, foods eaten, places visited outside the home, exposure to pollens, weather conditions. Add anything you feel may contribute to the asthma. Then keep a note of when your child comes into contact with or does anything on your list of suspects, and if there is any worsening of her asthma symptoms.
- If you suspect a food allergy or intolerance, consult a dietitian, nutritionist or nutritional therapist, who will be able to pin down the allergen via an elimination diet or allergen test (*see* 'Getting Diet Right', on page 31).

▦ STOPPING SMOKING

Kicking the nicotine habit is one of the first steps any parent should take if she has a child with asthma. Research consistently shows that living in an environment where someone smokes can trigger asthma or make it worse if it already exists. There is no doubt that giving up now will help your child immeasurably, as well as having many benefits for you.

Smoking counsellors maintain that, although aids like nicotine patches, acupuncture and hypnotherapy can help, the key to quitting smoking for good is *to want to stop*. The people who stop smoking and stay stopped are those who are highly motivated to do so. It stands to reason that, if you have a child with asthma, you are highly motivated to ease her symptoms, so you will also be well motivated to stop smoking!

In addition to this, there are plenty of other benefits which are well worth writing down and pinning somewhere prominent as a constant reminder of the reasons why it is good to give up. Reasons can range from fresher breath, more energy, increased fitness and money saved to reducing your risk of heart disease, stroke and many forms of cancer – and living longer.

Here are a few other tips for quitting.

- Plan ahead for the difficult times when your resistance is low. Know when you habitually like a cigarette, for instance first thing in the morning, after a meal, during a coffee break, or out socializing, and plan how you are going to handle these situations, what you are going to do. It may mean changing your usual routine; for example, going for a short jog first thing in the morning, working through your coffee break or getting straight up from the table after a meal.
- Do not think of giving up as a sacrifice. This is a negative path to walk because, in your worst moments, you will feel hard done by and give in. You are giving up because you want to give up, because you want the best for your child.
- Do not cut down, trying to give up gradually. It just leaves you

forever planning when you can have your next cigarette, so smoking is always on your mind.

• Fill your time so that you are not constantly thinking about cigarettes. You could use it as a motivation to get yourself fitter, catch up on chores or gardening, or spend more time with your child.

• Do something with the money you save by treating yourself every month. Money saved by not smoking soon mounts up and you will find you have enough for a considerable treat. And it will remind you how much money you burned before you gave up smoking.

Once you have given up, do not lose sight of all the benefits – keep your written list handy. Do not give in to other smokers and the 'just-one-won't-hurt' myth, and remind yourself frequently how much better your child's asthma is now she is not living in a smoky environment. That is something you have given her by giving up.

▨ CREATING A LOW-ALLERGEN HOME

No matter how well we clean, our homes are a paradise for house-dust mites. To fight the concentrations you will have to change your whole approach to interior decoration. Out go comfortable cushions, draping swathes of curtaining and thick-pile carpets, and in come vinyl or wood flooring, wooden or vinyl furniture and blinds at the windows. Some anti-house-dust mite strategies are extremely radical, so you will find two attack plans below: one is the deluxe, throw-out-and-start-again plan; the other is a scaled-down version for children with milder symptoms or for those who cannot make the wholesale changes of the first plan. But you can always mix and match between them, making changes where you can.

Here are a few tips before you start.

• Be sure that your child's asthma is affected by house-dust mites.

- Get any thoughts out of your mind that your home is dirty. House-dust mites inhabit any home, no matter how much you clean.
- Do not feel you are failing your child if you do not put all these tactics into action. This is a round-up of everything that may be helpful; you do not have to do it all. If you just keep your child's bedroom as mite-free as possible by following the tips here, you will be helping her asthma considerably.

The comprehensive strategy

This overhaul is for those waging war on house-dust mites, and calls for major changes and considerable expense!

- Remove all carpets from the house and replace them with hard-wood flooring or linoleum. If you use rugs, choose ones with a short weave which can be washed at 60°C (house-dust mites are killed off at this temperature), and vacuum them every day.
- Remove all curtains and replace them with blinds. Vertical blinds are the best anti-allergy alternative, as they do not encourage dust to settle.
- Replace upholstered furniture with leather, vinyl or plain wooden sofas and chairs. Put cushions in sealed anti-allergy covers, wash the outer covers regularly at 60°C, and vacuum every day.
- Replace divan beds with wooden-framed beds and put the mattresses in sealed covers. Dispose of padded headboards. If your child sleeps in a bunk bed, put her in the top bunk, as house-dust mite droppings come through the mattress.
- Put sealed covers around your child's bedding (duvet, pillows) and wipe them down every week; although house-dust mites cannot get through the covers to the bedding or mattress, they build up on the surface.
- Wash your child's bedlinen every week at 60°C and dry in a hot dryer; on warm days, dry it outside (as long as pollen is not a trigger for your child's asthma – *see* pages 29–31). If possible, clothes should also be washed at 60°C.

- Radiators are great dust-gatherers: use the thinnest radiators available and damp-dust them regularly.
- Washing machines create a lot of lint and dust so move yours out of the house into the garage or an outhouse. If this is not possible, do the washing in a little-used room with the door closed.
- Use electricity for cooking rather than gas.
- Cut down on dust-gatherers around the home – books and book shelves, lampshades and standard lamps, ornaments, picture frames, plants and toys. Even textured wallpaper harbours dust! It need not be quite as drastic as it sounds: toys can be kept in a cupboard rather than a toy box; ornaments and books can be put behind glass in a cabinet; pictures can be put into flat clip frames which do not gather the same amount of dust as those with a raised border.
- If you live in a centrally heated home, keep your child's bedroom cool and do not let temperatures in the rest of the house to get too high.
- If possible try to dust with a damp cloth and vacuum the house every day. Do the housework when your child is not around, as it puts dust and allergens into the air while it is being done.
- Make sure you have good air circulation in your home, so that there is no build-up of gases, fumes, pollens and dust, and so that humidity levels are comfortable. If you have a chimney, open the fireplace up – make a decorative feature of it if there is no solid-fuel fire in it. Keep a window open upstairs and one downstairs to encourage air circulation and always open a window after using chemical household liquids, bleaches, cleaning fluids, etc. Do not block up air bricks.
- Do not let the air become too humid as this can encourage damp and cause asthma symptoms in some people. Dry clothes outdoors or in a tumble dryer. Open windows in steamy rooms like bathrooms or fit an extractor fan. Keep plants out of the house as they encourage humidity as well as harbouring dust.

The scaled-down strategy

This approach is not as radical as the previous plan, but it does involve considerable, dedicated hard work.

- Make all the changes suggested above, but just to your child's bedroom: remove carpets and curtains; change the bed; put sealed covers on the mattress and bedding and wipe these down regularly; wash outer bedding every week at 60°C and dry it outside or in a hot dryer; and remove as many dust-gatherers as possible. Damp-dust and vacuum the room every day.
- Dispose of dust-gatherers in the rest of the house.
- If possible, damp-dust and vacuum the rest of the house every day when your child is not around.
- Put the tips on air circulation and humidity levels suggested above into practice.

Toys

Furry and fabric toys harbour house-dust mites which means you will have to rethink your child's toy collection if mites are a trigger for her asthma.

- Avoid soft, cuddly, furry or fabric toys as these are ideal breeding grounds for house-dust mites and can cause maximum aggravation for the child, as they are likely to be held close, cuddled and slept with. You need to be drastic: let your child keep her favourite cuddly toys, then dispose of the rest.
- Favourite cuddlies need careful attention: put them in the freezer in a plastic bag overnight, once a week, to kill off the mites; then wash them at 60°C.
- Also avoid fabric story books, fabric bricks, a dressing-up box and anything which might provide a home for dust. Stick to plastic or wooden toys. Wash dolls' clothes regularly at 60°C.
- Do not store toys where they can gather dust; put them in a closed drawer or cupboard, sort them out regularly and wash them if they seem to be getting dusty.

Buying specialist equipment

If you have a child with asthma then you will not have missed the many advertisements for specialist home equipment. These products range from full house-dust mite eradication to air filters and vacuum cleaners. Some make rather grandiose health claims for their products and the National Asthma Campaign and the Consumers' Association in the UK have accused some manufacturers of exploiting parents' fears about their children's health. However, some *may* make a difference in some instances. If you are considering buying one, weigh up the possible benefits to your child against the outlay, bearing in mind what you believe to be the triggers of her asthma.

• **Anti-allergy bedding/sealed covers.** Anti-allergy bedding is duvets and pillows which come 'sealed' so that house-dust mites cannot get through. Sealed covers are designed to go over ordinary mattresses, pillows and duvets to stop house-dust mites getting through. They are now widely available and the price has come down somewhat since they first came on the market. They are effective at keeping mite levels low in the bed; however, you have to be vigilant in the rest of the bedroom for them to make a great difference.

• **Anti-allergy vacuum cleaners.** Regular vacuum cleaners send a lot of dust back into the air; anti-allergy versions contain a special filter which draws the dust into the cleaner, where it is sealed in place; there are also vacuum cleaners designed to pick up more pet hairs. There are obvious advantages in cutting down on the movement of dust in the home if it is a trigger for asthma. However, it is difficult to know how good a lot of these cleaners are and whether they live up to the manufacturer's claims. Your best bet if you want to buy one (and they are not cheap) is to look for one which comes with an independent seal of approval such as endorsement by an organization like the British Allergy Foundation.

• **Ionizers and air purifiers.** Ionizers produce negative ions which attach themselves to particles like dust and pollen and draw them out of the air. In tests, they have not shown themselves to be very effective in helping with asthma, although some hay fever sufferers find they can ease the symptoms. Another product linked to asthma is a vaporizer, which burns decongestant oils like menthol and eucalyptus which obviously help to clear congested bronchial passages but would not stop an asthma attack.

- **Air filters.** These can help filter allergen particles out of the air, but will not eradicate them completely, since dust is mobilized every time we move, so more is constantly thrown into the air. If you do buy one (and they are expensive), opt for a high-efficiency particle air (HEPA) filter.

- **House-dust mite extermination.** You can either do this yourself by buying an acaricide which kills the mite, or get someone to come to your home and do it for you. However, it is virtually impossible to rid your home of house-dust mites entirely or for good; they multiply too quickly and are too resilient to be beaten this way. A 1997 study conducted at Tel Aviv University in Israel, and featuring 46 allergic asthmatic children, compared using an acaricide plus house-dust mite avoidance measures with using house-dust mite avoidance measures alone. The results showed that the acaricide made no difference to children's symptoms at all, although house-dust mite avoidance measures (the tactics outlined above) were a significant help.

PETS

Like favourite cuddly toys, the problem of a family pet is one many of us try to put off, even though we know the animal makes our child's asthma symptoms worse. It is easy to say 'Get rid of pets', but we become very attached to them. If a pet is old, it may be difficult to find it a new home and then the alternative is to have it put down.

Case Study
'I knew once we had made the connection between Nicola's asthma and animals, that we would have to get rid of the cat,'

remembers Lisa. 'But Nicola loved it – Pixie had been with us since before Nicola was born so she'd grown up with it. So we postponed finding it a new home until it became obvious that the asthma wouldn't improve while the cat was in the house. Now, I'm glad we did it because Nicola is so much better, although she still has to be careful at friends' houses.'

We do tend to put our pets before our health: a Canadian study of nearly 350 patients allergic to dogs or cats, reported in the *British Medical Journal,* found that only one in five of the patients followed medical advice and got rid of their pets; around three-quarters even replaced an animal that had died with a new pet.

If your pet is a trigger for your child's asthma, you have a choice: you can find a new home for it, or keep it but be prepared to work hard to keep irritant levels as low as possible. This means:

- brushing it every day, outside the house or when your child is not present
- bathing it once a week in a good insecticidal shampoo – ask your vet to recommend a brand – which can remove quite a lot of the dander (fur and hair) that causes irritation
- not letting it onto upholstered furniture – certainly not in bedrooms and on beds.

Brushing, bathing and training a dog may not be too difficult (although I have not come across many dogs who enjoy a bath); cats are a different matter. If you have the animal from a kitten, start the brushing and bathing programme at once and it will not know any different. With an older cat, wear protective gloves!

BEATING THE POLLEN COUNT

If your child's asthma is affected by pollen, you are in for a tough spring and summer, as asthma symptoms combine with those of hay fever (runny nose and eyes, tickly throat, itchy skin). It makes sense to lower the amount of pollen she comes into contact with, even if you cannot avoid it completely.

You can start by making your garden as low-allergen as possible. The British National Asthma Campaign (NAC) created a low-allergen, low-maintenance garden for the Chelsea Flower Show in 1996: low-allergen to help people whose asthma is triggered by pollens and low-maintenance to help those whose asthma is exacerbated by physical exertion. Most of the tips incorporated into it can be put into action in your own garden.

• Grass produces pollens, so cut back on your lawn with paving and patio areas; do not mow it when your child is around.
• Plant insect-pollinated plants rather than wind-pollinated ones, which reseed themselves by casting their pollens into the air; insect-pollinated varieties are stickier and heavier, and rely on insects to carry the pollen with them. Ask your garden centre to show you which are which.
• Avoid plants which are heavily scented, as these can irritate sensitive airways.
• Opt for fences and walls in place of hedges, which are traps for pollens and mould spores.
• Cut down on weeds by putting down a good layer of gravel mulch or planting ground-cover plants.
• Do not start a compost heap, as these harbour mould spores.

The problem with a low-allergen garden is that it is not very child-friendly, as it is a rather bare, paved environment; the NAC suggests pots and garden ornaments to fill spaces, but ornaments and young children are not perfect partners.

It is also true that, no matter how much you labour to make your own garden low in pollens, there is not much you can do about your neighbours' and pollens can be carried some distance. Trees, parks and even planted traffic islands can also be sources of wind-borne pollens. However, having a relatively pollen-free area on the doorstep may mean the difference between your child spending time in the garden and staying indoors with the windows closed.

Here are some additional tips for the high-pollen season:

- If you want your child to be outside, encourage her to spend time in the garden in the early morning or late evening, as pollen counts are lowest at these times.
- Do not bring flowers or plants from outside into the house; even if they are not wind-pollinated varieties, they may still have pollen clinging to them from other plants.
- Do not dry clothes outside during the high-pollen season, since wind-borne pollens can settle on clothing.
- Keep dogs and cats well brushed. Animals brush against plants and roll in grass all the time and pollen clings to fur. Brush them outside the house.
- Keep windows shut in the daytime; open them in the early morning or late evening, or after rain, to let in fresh air.
- If mould pollens are a problem for your child, keep an eye out for any dampness in the house. Treat damp areas and keep them clean so that they do not develop the characteristic 'spotting' of mould. Make sure that steamy areas – bathroom and kitchen – have good ventilation.

GETTING DIET RIGHT

We are only just beginning to realize how important diet is to children's health and development, as a growing bank of research links dietary deficiencies with a range of growth, developmental and behavioural problems. Recently, more interest has focused on diet and its relationship with asthma. Certain vitamins and minerals have been shown to help alleviate the symptoms (*see* box on pages 36–7), although it is a leap from this to proving that deficiencies trigger asthma. It has also been suggested that changes in the Western diet could play a part. Research done at Auckland Hospital in New Zealand, for example, found a link between the rise in asthma and the move away from eating animal fats. Other research has found that:

- Breastfeeding for at least the first six months can protect against the development of asthma. Allergic conditions like asthma and eczema are estimated to be seven times more common in formula-fed babies than those who are breastfed. The protective factor in breast milk is thought to be the high levels of antibodies it contains, which provide the intestine wall with a protective lining in the early days after the birth. Babies on formula milk miss out on these antibodies while formula introduces foreign proteins into the immature intestine. It is these foreign particles which are thought to set up the allergic reaction which develops into a food allergy, asthma or eczema. In addition, the immune system (which is involved in the development of asthma) also has to cope with these foreign proteins at a time when it is most vulnerable.
- Past the baby stage, the best protective diet against asthma is one rich in antioxidant vitamins (vitamins C and E and betacarotene, the precursor to vitamin A). The best way to achieve an antioxidant-rich diet is to give your child a varied menu with plenty of fresh fruit and vegetables, lean meat and fish (particularly oily fish like mackerel, sardines and salmon) and starchy foods like bread, pasta, potatoes and rice. It is important to ensure that she gets adequate supplies of calcium, particularly if she has to take high doses of steroid medication, so build in lots of calcium-rich foods like dairy products and green, leafy vegetables, fish and pulses. Steroids are associated with an increased risk of osteoporosis later in life, where calcium leaches from the bones making them brittle and prone to fracture. Although the usually low doses taken in via an inhaler have not been associated with side-effects, it is still worth building up your child's calcium levels: it is in the first 20 years of life that bone mass is laid down, so good bone density now can protect against osteoporosis later.
- Additives in foods have been linked with asthma, so it makes sense to cut them out of your child's diet as much as possible.

Opting for the fresh-food diet outlined above will get you off on the right foot. Then take care with foods and drinks aimed at children and read the labels carefully. Possible links between pesticide residues in fresh produce and a whole raft of illnesses from ME to asthma indicate that buying organic produce where possible will also help your child.

Building a healthy diet
Beyond the weaning stage, a healthy, basic diet for children and teenagers is not very different from an adult's. Your child should eat a good variety – not always easy if you have a fussy toddler. Try not to worry if she goes through phases of being fussy (no toddler ever starved herself) and work towards including some foods from each of the following groups every day:

- fresh or frozen fruit and vegetables, particularly green leafy vegetables, carrots, citrus fruits and salads
- meat and fish; eggs (well cooked to avoid salmonella poisoning)
- starchy foods like bread, potatoes, pasta, rice and breakfast cereals
- beans, lentils and other pulses
- dairy foods (milk, cheese, yoghurt, fromage frais).

With dairy and wheat-based foods, watch out for allergic reactions or intolerances which may be exacerbating the asthma, and seek guidance from a dietitian or nutritional therapist.
Be sparing with:

- sweets and sweet things, including sweetened and fizzy drinks
- salt (no salt under one year)
- fatty foods like processed convenience meals, fried foods and fatty snacks
- processed foods which contain a lot of additives

Do not give a preschool child nuts, unless they are ground, as there is a risk of choking; nuts are also a common cause of allergic reactions.
For more advice on weaning, *see* chapter 6.

Is it a food allergy or intolerance?

It is not always simple to find out if your child's asthma is triggered by a food or foods, unless there is an immediate reaction, in which case your child has an allergy rather than an intolerance. In the majority of cases, however, a child will have an intolerance and in these instances it takes time for a reaction to show up, so you may not make the link between the food and the asthma symptoms. In addition, the most common allergens are wheat and dairy products, which are generally the mainstay of a child's diet and thus eaten too often for a link to stand out.

Suspect a food intolerance if any of the following applies.

• There is a history of food intolerance in the family.
• You have noticed an association between eating a certain food and the later development of asthma symptoms. If you really want to tie this down, keep a food diary for a month, noting what foods your child eats every day and any changes or worsening of asthma symptoms. Over a few weeks, you should see a pattern emerging. You may find the food responsible is a particular favourite of your child's – we appear to crave the thing which makes us ill!
• Your child has other symptoms associated with an intolerance, for example frequent diarrhoea or constipation, bloated stomach, eczema, shadows under eyes, general lethargy and recurrent infections.

Case Study

'Both William and I have asthma,' says Monica (William's mother), 'but I didn't make the connection between it and food for a long time. I actually went to see a nutritional therapist about a stubborn weight problem and the therapist did some tests and told me I had an intolerance to dairy products. When they were knocked out of my diet, not only did my weight go down as my energy levels went up, but my asthma symptoms cleared. I thought maybe William's asthma might be caused by dairy products as well so he went along for an assessment and sure enough, the tests showed up an allergic reaction. We removed dairy products from his diet and his asthma also improved. It hasn't gone completely – he tends to get symptoms in the spring and summer, when the pollen's high – but he certainly doesn't get it all year round now.'

If you suspect an intolerance, the next step is to consult your doctor, who can refer you to a dietitian, or else see a nutritional therapist privately. Nutritional therapists are complementary practitioners who use diet to overcome health problems and are trained to track down and treat food intolerances. (For more on nutritional therapy, *see* chapter 5.)

Although there are a number of tests available which can help pinpoint a food allergen, the most conclusive way is via an elimination diet, which reduces what you eat to a few foods – usually pears, rice and lamb, which do not appear to prompt allergic reactions. After four days, other foods are reintroduced, one food group at a time, to see if there is a reaction. Your child's elimination diet will probably last four weeks, although she may be put on a preliminary diet featuring fresh, whole foods to get her digestive system up to par. If she does have a food intolerance, she will go through these stages on an elimination diet:

1 food-withdrawal, when she will feel lethargic and flu-like, possibly craving the food causing the problems; this stage lasts for around three to four days, while the food leaves the body
2 improvement, when she should start to feel much healthier, with more energy and fewer or no asthma symptoms
3 the challenge, when foods are reintroduced; you will need to keep a food diary at this stage to note any return of symptoms and foods eaten

Common foods causing allergies or intolerances in children
- dairy products (milk, including formula, cheese, butter, yoghurt, etc)
- wheat products (specifically the protein gluten in wheat): bread, cakes, biscuits, cereals, etc
- eggs
- citrus fruits
- tomatoes
- yeast
- sugar
- soya products (including soya-based formula)
- food additives

- chocolate
- nuts, including peanut butter and peanut oil – if your child has a peanut allergy, be extra vigilant as peanut oil is a hidden extra in many processed foods and snacks

Once a food intolerance has been established, your dietitian or nutritional therapist will help you to work out a suitable diet for your child. The guilty foods will not necessarily be completely forbidden: many people find that eating the foods in rotation – that is, only eating them once within, say four days or a week – helps them avoid reaching their allergen threshold.

Some children may be intolerant to a number of foods, which can make keeping your child to a healthy diet difficult. Being on an elimination diet can be restricting, particularly if there is a long list of suspect foods and they include staples like wheat and dairy products. For these reasons, it is vital to go to someone experienced in food intolerance diagnosis; some doctors take an interest in it, but in general medical practice it is largely the province of dietitians. There are also specialist allergy clinics in some areas to which your doctor may refer you, as well as nutritional therapists. Growing children need a healthy, balanced diet, particularly if they are fighting a condition like asthma, and their immune system should be in fighting-fit form. Excluding foods could lead to nutritional deficiencies which may cause harm in the long run, which is why it is not advisable for you to put your child on an elimination diet without professional guidance.

Vitamin and mineral help
Some vitamins and minerals appear to help alleviate the symptoms of asthma. However, most of the studies involved used therapeutic doses of the nutrient taken as supplements rather than foods and *you should not give your child supplements without professional guidance*. A child's nutrient needs are different from an adult's and supplementation carries a risk of overdosing.

Building foods rich in these nutrients into your child's diet is risk-free, so try that avenue first. If you want to take it further, consult a nutritional therapist, who will assess your child individually to see if her levels of these nutrients need increasing.

- **Antioxidant vitamins A (as betacarotene), C and E.** Low levels of A and C have been associated with increased wheezing and breathlessness. A number of trials link vitamin C with a reduction in asthma symptoms, and vitamin C levels in people with asthma are often lower than in non-asthmatics. In one study, taking 2g of ascorbic acid (vitamin C) before exercise helped protect against exercise-induced asthma.
  Sources: betacarotene: carrots, parsley, green leafy vegetables like spinach, spring greens and watercress, tomatoes, cantaloupe melon; vitamin C: blackcurrants, strawberries, citrus fruits, parsley, green leafy vegetables; vitamin E: vegetable oils, almonds, wheatgerm, cod liver oil, peanut butter.
- **Vitamin B6 (pyridoxine).** Some asthmatics appear to have a deficiency in B6 and anti-asthma drugs like theophylline can make it worse. In an American study, children with moderate to severe asthma were given 200mg of B6 daily for five months and experienced fewer symptoms and asthma attacks and needed less medication than a comparison group not taking B6. Another study shows an improvement with 50mg of B6, twice a day.
  Sources: wheatgerm, oats, yeast extract, liver, potatoes, bananas.
- **Magnesium.** A 1985 clinical trial found this mineral to have a significant effect on lung function in people with asthma. Another study has shown that magnesium, given intravenously, can improve pulmonary function and reduce the time in hospital after an attack.
  Sources: Nuts, yeast extract, wholemeal bread, brown rice, bananas, peas.
- **Polyunsaturated fatty acids (PUFAs).** A 1997 study at the University of Wyoming found that a moderate amount of PUFAs in the diet could improve symptoms in mild cases of asthma.
  Sources: oily fish like mackerel, sardines, fresh tuna, trout and salmon.

Chapter Three

The Emotional Aspects of Asthma

Amid all the suggestions for practical change, no one should lose sight of the fact that rising above asthma is also about handling the emotional ups and downs. There are three main aspects to this emotional and psychological side. First, asthma can be brought on by stress, tension and other emotions, so children need to be shown ways of handling stress in their lives. Secondly, children themselves have feelings and worries about being asthmatic that they may need help to understand, come to terms with or simply keep in proportion. And thirdly, there are parents, who often experience – and have to learn to handle – a range of emotions relating to the fact that their child has asthma, which can range from stress when he has a return of asthma symptoms or an attack to a fear of having to care for a child with so chronic a condition. It is important to acknowledge these feelings and seek help to overcome them if necessary, because the way your child feels about having asthma – and the way *you* feel about it – translates directly into how well he handles the condition and lives a normal life despite it.

▨ FIGHTING STRESS, EASING ANXIETY

Both asthmatic children and their parents are bound to feel the effects of stress and anxiety: stress because it is so much a part of the way we live nowadays, and anxiety because it is very hard not to be anxious if there is someone with asthma in the family. It may not be a constant anxiety, but it can erupt each time there is a worsening of symptoms or the likelihood of an attack. If a child's asthma is triggered by stress, then a vicious circle can develop. If he encounters a stressful situation, he may become anxious that it will bring on an asthma attack, which in turn adds to his stress levels and increases the likelihood of asthma symptoms developing. In addition, although asthma is by no means all in the mind, emotions like anxiety, depression and unhappiness can undoubtedly exacerbate the symptoms.

Because stress and anxiety play such a role in asthma, it is helpful to have strategies for handling them. The ones outlined below can work for both adults and children, although you will have to adapt them to your child's age and understanding. They should be practised when your child is not having an asthma attack but once mastered they will not only help him deal with stress and anxiety, but also have the knock-on effect of helping him to cope during an attack.

Posture

The way we hold ourselves gives a good indication of whether we are feeling stressed or anxious (hunched shoulders, stiff neck, clenched jaw). Simply by relaxing and improving our posture, we can lessen these feelings. A condition like asthma can also cause your child to become tensed, particularly around the shoulders, neck and upper back, as he copes with his breathing difficulties. But by tensing this area he is making his lungs work harder; by correcting his posture and loosening up, he will open up his lung cavity, giving the lungs room to breathe and helping the diaphragm work efficiently – all of which could help ease his symptoms.

A simple posture exercise is to stand with your feet slightly apart, and imagine you have a piece of string running through your body, coming out of the middle of your head. Now imagine someone pulling the string up from your head so that your whole body rises and straightens. Pull in your stomach, keep your back straight (not arched) and shoulders down and slightly back. Position your head in the centre of your neck and have your chin at right angles to your neck. This is a posturally correct stance.

Of course, keeping this up is practically impossible without a lot of practice. Learning a posturally balanced health programme like the Alexander technique, Pilates or yoga can help good posture become a way of life. A relaxation session (*see* below) at least once a day is a way to make you or your child more aware of the tension in the body, as well as how to get rid of it. Certainly, the least you should do when you are under pressure or feeling overanxious is check your posture through the day and consciously relax tensed areas.

Relaxation

Relaxation techniques are a well-tested and validated means of letting go of stress and anxiety, combining physical muscle relaxation with focused mental relaxation. You start by losing tension from your body before moving on to lowering levels of mental stress through visualization. All it takes is a commitment to put aside at least 20 minutes a day, every day, although two sessions a day is even more productive.

In 'Your relaxation programme' (*see* box opposite), you will find a basic guide to relaxation techniques. Alternatively, there is a good selection of relaxation tapes available from bookshops and health stores which guide you through a prerecorded routine; these usually include a muscle relaxation programme and a mental visualization accompanied by calming music or sounds. Although they are based on hypnotherapy techniques, there is no worry about you or your child losing control or 'going under'. The process is very gentle. It works around you, allowing you to let go, and is completely safe for most people. (Consult your doctor before using a relaxation tape, however, if you suffer from epilepsy.)

A visualization is simply a calming scenario to help you relax. It can be a generalized calming scene – for example, lying on a tropical beach listening to the waves, lying on warm grass beside a stream with the sun touching your face, walking through a wood along a winding path with the scent of pine around you, listening to the birds or lying watching the clouds. Alternatively, you can call up somewhere peaceful you have been before, where you were calm and happy, and hold that scene in your mind. As you go through the visualization, do not worry if thoughts intrude; just let them skate across your mind and then let go of them.

With your help, your child can also try visualization. At its most simple, ask him to imagine a happy place and fill it with favourite things: pets, sunshine, sea, grassy hills, flowers, birds. Perhaps you could ask him to imagine he is walking along a beach, feeling the sand in his toes, listening to the sea and the seagulls, or walking along a winding path through a beautiful garden, full of butterflies, turning a corner and finding a little house, opening the door, and so on.

It takes a little practice but, if it is done regularly, you will find that relaxation and visualization become easier and you let go more readily, so a quick five- or ten-minute relaxation session two or three times a day can refresh you. If you are a beginner at this type of relaxation process, find a quiet room in the house where you can lie down and not be disturbed; make sure it is warm and you are wearing loose, comfortable clothing. Once you become used to it, however, you and your child should be able to go through the process anywhere, for instant stress release.

Your relaxation programme
1 Lie down somewhere comfortable and close your eyes. Focus on your breathing: breathe in through your nose and take the breath down into your stomach. Feel your stomach rise as you inhale and fall as you exhale. Breathe slowly and regularly.
2 Starting at your feet, tense or squeeze your muscles for five seconds and then let go and relax them for 10–15 seconds. Slowly move up your body (legs, stomach, back, shoulders/neck, arms and face), tensing or squeezing the muscles in each area for five seconds, then relaxing them for around ten seconds before moving on. If your child finds it difficult to squeeze certain areas of his body (ie back, shoulders), go on to the next area.

3 Tense your whole body, hold for five seconds then let it all go.
4 Go through your body, checking for any remaining areas of tension, and follow the tense-relax programme again if you find any.
5 Visualize yourself somewhere peaceful and happy and allow your mind to relax. Do not chase any thoughts that enter your mind; let them go and continue with your visualization.
6 When you feel ready and totally relaxed, refocus on your breathing and open your eyes. Get up slowly and give your body a good stretch to end the relaxation exercise.

Breathing

When we are under stress or overanxious, we tend to breathe quickly and shallowly. There is a good reason for this: feeling stressed prompts our primitive 'flight or fight' response and the body gears up either to fight a perceived danger or to run away from it; either way, it will need more oxygen to turn into energy and overbreathing in this way brings more oxygen into the body. However, a prolonged episode of this type of breathing leads to hyperventilation, where the balance of oxygen and carbon dioxide in the body is upset, causing a range of symptoms: breathing difficulties, tight chest or chest pains, trembling, tingling, dizziness and lethargy. In fact, the symptoms of hyperventilation are similar to those of an asthma attack and obviously if a child hyperventilates during an attack, it will make the asthma symptoms worse.

If you or your child tend to overbreathe under stress, you need to practise slowing down your breathing. The following exercise will help:

1 Exhale as much stale air from your lungs as possible by giving a long, sighing out breath.
2 With one hand on your stomach, breathe in through your nose and let the breath go down to your stomach. You should feel your stomach rise.
3 Hold for a few seconds and let the breath go slowly out through your nose. One breathing cycle should take around eight seconds. If an eight-second cycle feels uncomfortable, start with a five-second cycle and build up to eight seconds as you practise.

Panic and asthma attacks

When symptoms of an asthma attack start (wheezing, coughing, difficulty breathing), many children panic. It is of course a natural reaction but it can create a vicious circle. Someone labouring to breathe tends to breath too fast or hyperventilate, which upsets the balance of oxygen and carbon dioxide in the blood at a time when oxygen is already having problems getting into the bloodstream. If your child tends to panic when asthma symptoms develop, try the following procedure:

- Stay calm yourself (or at least, stay outwardly calm); your child will feed off your panic.
- Slow down his breathing if he is overbreathing (quick, shallow, gasping breaths). Try the breathing exercise described opposite.
- Try to distract him away from worrying about his breathing. Ask him to count something around you (tiles on the walls, cars passing, books on the shelf, etc) or work out simple sums or spellings. Talk to him about something pleasant (a school trip, a holiday, the family pet) or go through a short visualization with him (*see* page 41).
- Try to damp down his anxiety. Panic attacks occur because of what is called 'anticipatory anxiety', where you envisage the worst. Help him break the negative pattern by concentrating on the positive steps you can take to overcome his asthma symptoms. Go through the management plan with him, talk to him about episodes when an asthma attack has been averted, describe all the weapons you have in your asthma arsenal, reassure him that it is not a bad attack.
- Talk to him again once the attack has stabilized and he is not upset or panicky, going over all the steps you can take, the ways you can help asthma symptoms, to reassure him and give him something to draw on next time an attack occurs.

Complementary therapies

Complementary therapies are good for handling stress and anxiety as well as helping with other emotional problems like depression or inability to cope. This is because they have a holistic approach to health, placing as much emphasis on how you feel emotionally as on how you feel physically. A complementary therapist would give greater significance to the effect of stress and anxiety on asthma symptoms than a conventional doctor.

Not to be undervalued, too, is the therapeutic value of just seeing a complementary therapist and spending a relaxed appointment simply talking. It is no coincidence that more and more complementary therapists also have qualifications in counselling.

Case Study

'I felt wonderful after I came away from my first appointment with my homeopath and I hadn't even taken a remedy,' says Pippa, 'because I'd spent one and a half hours talking about me. At some point, Matty's asthma came into it and I got a lot off my chest telling her about my worries. I found that in itself very therapeutic. I sort of rediscovered myself and got back my sense of perspective.'

Particularly recommended for tackling the emotional problems associated with asthma are homeopathy, Chinese medicine (including acupuncture) and reflexology. Studies have also shown hypnotherapy to be particularly successful in cases of asthma where there is an emotional trigger. Complementary therapies are also great stress-busters, particularly massage, meditation, aromatherapy, reflexology, yoga and the gentle Chinese movement art of t'ai chi. For more on complementary therapies, see chapter 5.

Beat stress

If being stressed is becoming a way of life for you or your child, take steps to make your environment and working life as stress-free as possible.

- Do not say yes to people when you really have not got the time to do the task (and that includes the family as much as work colleagues or schoolfriends). Delegate jobs or tasks where possible.
- Avoid 'multi-tasking', do one thing at a time. Juggling a lot of tasks stimulates the stress reaction in our bodies, which is just what you want to lower.
- De-stimulate your home environment to bring a little calm into your home life. Go for calming, pastel colours in your decor.

Turn down the TV or radio (even better, turn the TV off!) and keep noise levels in the home low – for example, do not have numerous appliances (washing machine, vacuum cleaner, blender) *and* the TV on at the same time. Employ subtle lighting – uplighters, lamps, candles – for evening relaxation.

• Stick to a healthy balanced diet and avoid quick-fix, high-sugar energy boosters, as these upset blood sugar levels and add to the body's stress burden. Avoid coffee, tea, alcohol and other stimulants.
• Take exercise. It releases pent-up energy (something children often need!), gives you a break from stressful situations and makes you feel good about yourself.
• Make time for yourself every day and be selfish with the time – do something you really want to do, *not* unfinished chores or homework.

THINKING POSITIVELY ABOUT ASTHMA

It is easy with asthma to fall into negative thinking, and envisage the worst-case scenario if your child develops symptoms or has an attack. Even if he is symptom-free, there is always the temptation to dwell on the next episode or attack. But this kind of thinking is not very helpful: if symptoms worsen or an attack occurs, you need to be able to think calmly and rationally to judge whether treatment is working or not, whether to move on to the next stage in your child's management plan, or whether to call for emergency help. When he is free of symptoms, you need to be able to get on with life without the nagging worry that another episode is on the horizon.

If you find yourself caught in a downward spiral, make an effort to promote the positive. Think about what you have on your side:

• My child's asthma is well controlled with medication and complementary treatment.
• I know what to do if symptoms develop or get worse.
• I know the signs of an imminent attack and I can take steps to avert it.

- I know what to do in the event of an attack.
- My child is strong and healthy.
- Emergency help is only a few minutes away.
- Fatal asthma attacks are rare in children.

Positive thinking stretches beyond the incidence of asthma episodes or attacks into your general attitude towards your child and his limitations. Instead of dwelling on the activities asthma stops your child doing, count those he can do. Do not think of how much time he has lost at school; consider ways to encourage him to catch up. In this way, you will move from a 'he can't' standpoint to a more motivational 'he can' view of your child and this attitude will filter through to him, lessening his anxieties, helping him cope better when he has asthma and spread his wings a bit when he does not.

Case Study

For Peta, mother to 11-year-old Peter, it was Peter himself who made her change her attitude. 'Peter's asthma is quite seasonal: he gets it in winter when it's very cold and also in the summer, when the pollen's about. But I worry the whole year round. I didn't realize it but I was stopping him from doing things when really there was no need. Then one day Peter asked if he could go the park with some friends. I automatically said he couldn't because it was cold out. He just said to me 'I can, Mum. I know I can.' For him, there was no reason about it being a problem. So I let him go and he was fine. Now, I question myself before I trot out 'You can't.' Often I turn the decision over to him and he's very good; if he doesn't think he should go somewhere, he doesn't. But he is willing to push himself more than I was willing to push him.'

How children feel about asthma

Children of course have their own views on their asthma and they are not always the views parents think they have. Children are generally great copers and may hide some of their greater worries so as not to make their parents more anxious. But even young children have a range of concerns about their asthma.

A 1996 study, conducted at the University of Rochester in New York and reported in the journal *Paediatric Nursing*, looked specifically at children's perceptions of asthma, its impact on their lives and their worries. The researchers found that, overall, 54 per cent of the children worried a lot about asthma with 64 per cent saying that their lives were a lot different due to asthma. The main themes were symptoms and treatments ('It's hard to breathe', 'You wheeze, your chest starts hurting, you throw up'), what asthma stopped them from doing (the 'I can't' category) and the restrictions asthma placed on them 'I'm not allowed to play outside', 'I always wanted to be in the army but grown-ups with asthma don't get into the army'). Fear of dying during an attack was another general fear ('If I forget my inhaler and I have short breath, I could die', 'Sometimes I think I am just going to stop breathing and die or something').

The worries tended to fall into specific age groups, however. Younger children (six- to seven-year-olds) were primarily concerned with their symptoms and having to take medication; in middle childhood and early adolescence, 'I can't' and restrictions were foremost. The good news is that older teenagers (up to age 18) had accepted their condition and the emotional mood had changed to one of positive adaptation: 'You learn to appreciate the simple things like running and how to laugh.', 'It's made me take responsibility for my medicine', 'I don't really measure asthma in terms of good and bad; I just accept it as part of my life'.

Other studies, and what children themselves say, throw up other asthma worries, like being different. Once they start school, children want to fit in. Asthma can set a child apart for a number of reasons: it can stop him doing everything his classmates do; he may have to use an inhaler in school; and he may spend a lot of time off school, which does not help when it comes to making friends. 'I don't like using my inhaler at school,' admits one six-year-old. 'Everyone looks at me.' On top of this, myths about asthma still abound and these colour other children's perception of the condition and the person who has it. These myths include an asthmatic child being 'weak' or 'putting it on' for attention, even that asthma is catching.

A feeling of not being good enough is also common. 'Asthma means I'm no good at games. I need my puffer or I just can't play,' said Darryl, a healthy ten-year-old with moderate but well-controlled asthma. 'I'm on the school netball team but I worry a lot about my asthma, that I might let everyone down when we're playing,' comments 12-year-old Sara, who has exercise-induced asthma.

Feeling as though they are not good enough and are different because of their asthma can lead to lowered self-esteem, so children constantly denigrate their achievements and lack confidence in themselves and what they can achieve. This is where parents have a strong role to play, in building up confidence and self-esteem and getting their child to face his fears and anxieties – and overcome them. The box below will give you some suggestions for building self-esteem. Even something as simple as telling your child to explain to his friends what asthma is can help take the mystique out of the condition; if he is having problems at school, it may mean arranging with the class teacher for an asthma expert to come in and have a chat with the children.

A parent's role is to help and encourage their child to think positively and realistically about asthma, capitalizing on what he can do, putting worries into perspective and showing the child how he can overcome or work round restrictions in his life. To do this, parents themselves need to be honest about their own feelings.

Building your child's self-esteem

Having asthma can knock your child's confidence, in that he may feel different from his classmates and sometimes feel left out because he cannot do all that his friends do. Parents need to bolster a child's self-esteem and confidence in himself and his abilities, and the following tips might help.

- As soon as you think your child will understand about his asthma, explain what it is and how it affects him, and stress that he has not got asthma because of something he did wrong. In this way, he will be able to come to terms with and accept his condition, and know what is happening when he does get an attack. It will also help him explain to others what asthma is.

- Give your child lots of avenues in life instead of focusing solely on one hobby or activity; in this way, he will see he has a range of abilities and, although he may not excel in one area, in others he can be the leader of the pack.
- Always build up the positives (what your child can do) rather than dwelling on the negatives (what he cannot do). Encourage him to accept what he cannot do and move on to something he can; explain that nothing is crucial – he can always go back to something he wants to do at a later date.
- Do your bit to avoid knocks in confidence. This is particularly important when your child starts school: make sure teachers know about his asthma, give clear instructions on what to do if he has an attack, and ensure that he always has his reliever inhaler with him.
- Try not to say 'no' all the time. Before snapping out a negative, weigh up whether something he wants to do *will* cause problems; take into consideration the fact that his asthma is well controlled, that he can take extra medication if necessary, even that his condition may have become milder over the years. If you decide the answer is still no, give him a good reason why you feel he should not do what he wants to.
- Let your child make some of the decisions in his life. Knowing you trust him is one of the best ways to build up his confidence. For a child with asthma, letting him take responsibility for his health care as soon as he can is a sure way of building self-esteem.

How parents feel about asthma

Having a child with asthma can stir up very mixed emotions in parents, which colour the way they view his condition, how they treat him and how well they take on the responsibilities that come with asthma. The most common feelings experienced by parents are:

- **Anxiety.** Being overanxious is the greatest emotional hurdle that parents have to overcome. Anyone who has been through an asthma attack will worry that his child will have another and any return of symptoms, however slight, brings with it those anxieties. And there is also the rarely mentioned fear that asthma can be fatal.

Case Study
'All the time I think I have it at the back of my mind. I know all the statistics and the odds, but it's still there,' admits Karen, mother of two boys, aged 4 and 7, who both have asthma.

'If he has an attack, I follow the procedure worked out with the clinic nurse, but actually all I want to do is bundle him into the car and race to the hospital,' says Patrick, father of six-year-old Nathan. 'I just want lots of experts there, in case something goes wrong.'

- **Guilt.** If one parent has brought the asthma tendency into the family (either if they have asthma themselves or if there is a strong family tendency towards it), then sometimes he feels guilty of passing it on or causing his child's asthma. In addition, parents also sometimes blame themselves for having done something, or not done something, which may have triggered it.

Case Study
'I always felt guilty that I didn't breastfeed Justin,' admits Barbara. 'I breastfed his sister and she is asthma-free. I changed Justin to the bottle at four weeks because I couldn't seem to satisfy him. I don't know if there is any link between the bottle-feeding and the asthma – Justin didn't develop asthma until he was two years old – but every time I read something about allergies and early feeding, I just feel I could have done better by Justin.'

- **Fear of responsibility.** Having someone with a chronic illness in the family brings responsibilities: for giving or taking medication, monitoring the condition, spotting signs that symptoms are worsening and making decisions during an attack. Sometimes, parents find it difficult to take on this responsibility. They themselves lack confidence in their own ability to spot changes in the condition, administer medication and support their child.

These feelings can lead to a number of problems, like over-protecting your child and overcompensating for his disabilities, wrapping him in cotton wool and not allowing him to take responsibility for his asthma care as he grows up. They may also make you put your own life on hold to look after your child, which can cause resentments to build up, particularly if one person feels he has done all the giving.

Parents' attitudes also dictate the balance of a family, something which is particularly important if there are other, non-asthmatic children in the family. Being overprotective or overcompensatory towards one child skews the family balance and puts pressure on brothers and sisters who do not have asthma and see their sibling being treated differently to them.

Case Study

'It seemed to me that Wayne was always let off things because of his asthma – chores, school, being yelled at,' remembers Tonia, thinking back to her childhood with an asthmatic brother. 'Mum more or less gave in to him every time and he got a lot more of her attention. I understand now it was because of his asthma – and the asthma was bad – but I really resented him.'

▦ WORKING IT OUT

There is a lot you can do yourself to overcome these emotional upheavals and keep a sense of perspective on the asthma, for both you and your child; the stress-relief measures outlined in the box on page 44–5 go a long way to controlling those inevitable anxieties.

You should also talk to your child about his asthma. Too often we concentrate on getting down to the practical day-to-day measures of asthma management without stopping to check how we are feeling about it inside. But being able to talk openly about worries, frustrations and even anger about asthma – and knowing that you are there to listen to him when he needs it – is vital for your child. Listening to your child also helps you to get your own worries into perspective.

Try to encourage your child to come forward with any worries from an early age, so that they can be sorted out promptly. Find out what symptoms bother your child most, what he worries about when he thinks about asthma, what he feels it stops him from doing. Once he is at school, you may need to look below the surface a little; children are very good at responding with a nonchalant 'OK' when asked if everything is all right, even when it is not. Focus on the positive, too: what he has achieved that he did not think he would be able to, how well the asthma is controlled, how steps you have taken in the home have helped his symptoms, what he can do for himself to keep symptoms away.

Worries about death can grow out of all proportion if they are not discussed and put into perspective. Children need to know that asthma can be life-threatening but that death from the condition is now, thankfully, very rare: around 1.5 million children have asthma in the UK but only around 30 of them die each year from the condition, and those will usually have asthma very severely. Statistics will not mean much to a young child, but they do allow you to reassure him that the chances of a fatal attack are microscopically low.

Reassure him in other ways, too. Let him know that you have a plan you follow when asthma symptoms come on. Talk through the management plan with him, so that he knows there is a routine to follow – routine is important and comforting to a young child. Emphasize how effective conventional and com-plementary treatments are at controlling asthma and how you are geared up to noticing changes in his symptoms and nipping them in the bud.

Encourage your child to lead as normal a life as possible, making allowances for his asthma but not allowing it to rule his life. Do not be afraid to push him a little, as you would a child without a chronic illness of this type: all children need a challenge, need to stretch themselves, and asthma should not be a bar to that.

Case Study

'Lee developed asthma at ten years old, probably brought on by exercise as it was discovered during a football match,' says Trudie. 'Being a keen sportsman, we hoped this wasn't going to interfere with the things he enjoyed doing most in life but he hasn't let it. He has got his asthma under control and has gone on to be player of the year for his town schools football league and plays football for his county. He has also come first in the 800 metres in his county.'

Do not treat him differently from his brothers and sisters. Let your child fight his own battles and earn his place in the family pecking order.

Finally, you need to admit when there are problems in the family that you cannot overcome or cope with, and seek professional help in sorting them out. Sometimes it may be too difficult to break the cycle of anxiety, stress and asthma on your own; or there may be problems within the family which call for outside assistance. Do not feel you have to muddle along if this is the case; many families which are learning to deal with a chronic illness have benefited from counselling; your doctor can refer you to a counsellor or you can seek one yourself (*see* 'Useful addresses' at the end of the book).

Family therapy, which involves the whole family, including brothers and sisters, has proved very helpful in cases of asthma. It can help to bring the family together and allows non-asthmatic brothers and sisters to gain a greater understanding of the problems faced by their asthmatic sibling and their parents. It also gives them a chance to voice their feelings about having asthma in the family. The approach is non-prescriptive: the counsellor may set goals for the family to achieve in specific problem areas, but by and large he acts as a facilitator, encouraging you to solve your own problems through better communication and understanding of each other's needs.

What is important in asthma, whether you seek counselling or not, is that you tackle it as a family and that no family member feels isolated; one parent should not feel the other has abandoned the responsibility of caring for their asthmatic child; no child with asthma should feel he has to cope with the problem without his parents' support; and brothers and sisters should not feel shut out because an asthmatic child appears to have a special relationship with a parent.

Although this book is largely concerned with the practicalities of having a child with asthma in the family, the emotional support and love he gets from his parents and brothers and sisters is as important as tracking down triggers. Growing up surrounded by a supportive, loving family ensures that a child is confident in his own ability to rise above the illness, become an independent individual, and live a full life.

Chapter Four

Conventional Treatments

There is presently no conventional cure for asthma, although progress is being made in tracking down a susceptibility gene which may lead to a cure in the future, or at least offer a way to spot children who are at higher risk of developing the condition and take protective steps before it has a chance to take hold. Until that time, we have a range of treatments which can control it quite effectively. On the one hand, there are anti-inflammatory drugs which help prevent the symptoms of asthma flaring up; on the other, there is a range of drugs called bronchodilators which act quickly in an attack to open airways. These two arms of asthma treatment have undoubtedly made it easier for children to live a normal life, participating in a way that asthma sufferers in previous generations were not able to do and allowing them to escape being regarded as 'delicate'.

These treatments can also be tailored to an individual's needs, which is important in an illness which varies so much from child to child and from episode to episode. Unless your child has severe asthma, this means that in the main her symptoms should be kept in check with a low dose. In mild cases, with only occasional asthma, your child may only have to use the relieving medication for quick control if symptoms develop.

■ CONTROLLING ASTHMA

Conventional treatment for asthma falls into two categories:

- preventers, which stop the symptoms from flaring up; your doctor will usually prescribe these to be taken every day, whether your child has symptoms or not
- relievers, which are used at the first signs of an attack, to stop the symptoms; they are also used when an attack is in progress.

Immunotherapy
Immunotherapy, which involves injecting the patient with a very diluted allergen solution which acts like a vaccine, neutralizing the allergy, is sometimes offered as a treatment for asthma. Because it carries a risk of prompting a severe asthma attack, however, it is now normally only carried out at specialist allergy clinics.

■ Preventers

These drugs work by preventing inflammation of the airways, thus stopping the other factors in the asthma equation (muscle spasm and mucus production) from kicking in. They come in various coloured inhalers, and include:

- corticosteroids (often simply called steroids), like beclomethasone, budesonide and fluticasone; if an attack is imminent, your child might also be prescribed prednisolone
- sodium cromoglycate or nedocromil, non-steroidal anti-inflammatory drugs
- salmeterol, a long-acting bronchodilator which can keep the airways open for up to 12 hours; at the moment it is usually prescribed in conjunction with steroids in severe cases of asthma.

■ Relievers

These drugs are called bronchodilators, because they open up constricted airways; they work quickly (within about 15 minutes) and their effect should last for four hours. They should only be used when your child actually has symptoms: they are her back-up for when regular preventive treatment fails to ward off an attack. They usually come in a blue inhaler. The most common types of reliever are:

- short-acting beta2-agonists, for example salbutamol and terbutaline, which are the first-line treatments in most cases
- ipratropium bromide which is often prescribed for very young children
- theophylline, a slow-release drug which may be prescribed if your child has more severe asthma or needs something to get her through the night; it has more side-effects than the other bronchodilators and needs careful monitoring by your doctor or clinic.

You know treatment is working when...
- your child is experiencing no – or minimal – symptoms
- there are no sudden deteriorations
- your child is only using her reliever occasionally, if at all
- your child's peak flow reading, if she is old enough to give one, comes in at 80 per cent or more of her best or predicted level, with only small daily variations
- there are no side-effects from medication
- she is able to live life to the full, including participating in sports

Your doctor will also be aiming to get your child to this level of health on the lowest dose of drugs possible without symptoms breaking through. She should reassess your child's progress regularly and make changes to treatment accordingly.

Taking medication

There are a number of ways your child can take her medication, but the preferred method is via inhalation. Since inhalers first came into use for asthma in the 1970s, they have revolutionized treatment by making medication more effective and localized, with a lower risk of side-effects. They are basically small hand-held devices which are put to the mouth as the drug is breathed in. The most common type is a *metered dose inhaler* (MDI or puffer, as it is often called), a pressurized aerosol which lets out a measured dose when you 'puff' it. However, MDIs are quite difficult for young children to use properly, because they demand quite a lot of co-ordination in learning how to puff and breathe in at the same time.

Even an MDI can be made simpler by the addition of a *spacer*, a cylinder which has a slot for the inhaler at one end and a mouthpiece at the other. The dose is puffed into the spacer and the child breathes it in. Getting a very young child to fasten her lips firmly round the mouthpiece can be difficult, however, so for those under two, you can use a spacer with a face mask. There are different types of spacer available, so talk to your doctor about which would be best for your child.

Using a spacer
This method is recommended for young children by the National Asthma Training Centre in the UK.

1 Remove the cap of the inhaler, give the inhaler a shake and insert it into the spacer.
2 Place the mouthpiece in your child's mouth, making sure there is a good seal; if you are using a face mask, place the mask over her face.
3 Ask her to breathe in and out steadily and gently; you will hear the spacer make a clicking noise as the valve opens and shuts.
4 Once she is breathing regularly, 'puff' the inhaler so that a single dose of medication enters the spacer.
5 Hold the spacer in place while the child breathes in and out five to eight times then remove it. Wait 30 seconds if another dose is needed.

Avoiding confrontation

Unless it tastes of strawberry and sugar, children can be remarkably resistant to taking medicine, and the paraphernalia that goes with asthma treatments – inhaler, spacer, mask – can be off-putting.

Case Study

'Matthew just could not master the inhaler, even with the spacer,' says Debra, a mother of two with a three-year-old asthmatic son. 'He didn't mind putting his mouth into the mask because I turned it into the "Magic Puff-Puff" game, all about a steam engine, which he loved – he was really into Thomas the Tank Engine at the time! The trouble was I was never sure he was breathing it in. I didn't hear the spacer click like it was supposed to so I spent a lot of time worrying he wasn't getting the medication into him. In the end, my doctor put him on syrup.'

Try to avoid confrontations, as they can turn every treatment time into a nightmare tussle. Here are some tips other parents have found helpful.

- Do not keep the inhaler and spacer a dark secret, only to be whipped out minutes before they are needed. Let your child touch and explore them, and leave them around the house where she can see them, so that they become familiar in an everyday setting – even if it means you have to wash them more frequently.
- With children under two especially, make sure your child feels secure when you give her medication. Hold her close in your arms, talk to her while you are giving the medication and look into her eyes. Try not to present a blank face. It is easy when you are trying to work an inhaler through a spacer to fall silent and have your face turned away, neither of which reassures a baby.
- With a baby, try to give the medication even if she cries. She will breath it in as she cries. Alternatively, hold the spacer and mask over her face as she sleeps.
- Try to pick a time of day when your child is most likely to be amenable. Avoid times when she is tired and irritable or has her mind on other things; she will not like being taken away from an absorbing game to be given medicine! Try not to give her her medication when you feel rushed or have an appointment

looming; inevitably, if you are in a hurry, the odds are your child will turn into a stubborn refusenik.

- Try to turn it into a game. Stick pictures on the spacer or decorate it; older children could be allowed to personalize it themselves. Debra turned it into a steam engine. Pretending to purr like kittens can also work. Another three-year-old was won round by pretending to be Darth Vader, complete with heavy breathing. Whatever works, as they say!

- If you attend an asthma clinic, a club or a support group, ask if your toddler can watch other children taking their medication. It helps to normalize the procedure and very often she will respond better to seeing another child using the equipment than to any amount of explaining and instruction from you.

- For persistent tantrum-throwers, a reward scheme may work. Avoid giving treats after each dose, however, as this can become a habit – and very quickly. Instead, start a star chart, where a star is added each time she takes her medicine without a fuss, and promise a non-sweet treat (such as a book or a small toy) if she attains a set number of stars in a week. You can gradually increase the number of stars she has to achieve before she is rewarded until, ideally, you are getting the full set each week. This is certainly worth the small outlay in treats.

- If giving medication has degenerated into a tussle, with tears and shouting on both sides, stop until you have both calmed down. Do something together, make an effort to show her that she is loved and secure, then try again a little later. Unless a toddler is having an asthma attack, it is more important to make her feel good about taking the medication than getting it into her at a set time.

- As soon as your child understands, try to explain to her how important it is that she takes her medication. Make the link early on between her symptoms and the fact that the medication will help her not to have those symptoms. Do not ram the message home or frighten your child with the dire consequences of not taking it, but go back to the conversation frequently. It is surprising how quickly children learn to take responsibility for their health once you make them aware of how they can help themselves.

If you do not feel your child is getting her medication because of difficulties in administering it or in using an inhaler, talk to your doctor about alternatives. Although she will be anxious for your child to get the hang of using a normal inhaler, she will also understand that young children are a special case. It may mean changing to a syrup or using a nebulizer for a while until she can master an inhaler. A nebulizer is a machine which is used in rare cases. It breaks down the liquid drug solution into a mist which the child breathes in via a face mask or mouthpiece. She does not have to learn a special technique to use it, but she must be willing to wear a face mask and sit still for ten minutes or so every time she has to take medication. A nebulizer is useful:

- for a child subject to 'brittle' asthma attacks – those that build from nothing to a critical point in a very short time, with no warning signs; having a nebulizer on hand to deliver high doses of reliever medication can be a lifesaver
- for a young child who cannot manage any of the inhalers on the market.

If you feel your child would benefit from a nebulizer, first discuss it with your doctor, as many health professionals have reservations about them for the following reasons:

- They make it difficult to measure dosage, as there are differences in nebulization rates, according to the drug used and the nebulizer.
- They are not portable – most run on electricity and are too unwieldy to carry around with you – which causes problems if reliever drugs are needed outside the home and neither you nor your child is practised at using an ordinary inhaler.
- You can get to rely on them too much so that you do not register when asthma is not being properly controlled by the medication, or when you should be seeking urgent assistance.

- They deliver a stronger dose of the drug solution, which raises the risk of side-effects.
- They stop a child from learning how to use an ordinary inhaler.
- They can cause hypoxia (deficiency of oxygen in the body), which is potentially fatal.

If your child is going to benefit fully from medication it is important that she feels comfortable with the type of inhaler she is using. Discuss inhaler options with your doctor, go back to her if you cannot get the hang of using it and ask to be shown how to use it if you are not offered a demonstration when medication is first prescribed.

Missing out on medication?

If your child is taking medication day in day out, it is easy to become careless. Research into the way asthma sufferers, including children, keep to their treatment plan has found that:

- Many people develop slipshod inhaler techniques, with the result that they do not get the right dose.
- Some people forget to take the medication. One American study found that, although around 95 per cent of children participating in the experiment said they had taken their medication as prescribed, in fact only around 58 per cent actually had.
- The patient or her parents fail to recognize when asthma is not being controlled by the drugs and the medication needs to move up a gear, either increasing the dosage or taking a short course of steroid tablets.

Pills and syrups

It is better to use the inhaled method of taking asthma drugs, for several reasons. Inhaling them means they go straight to the site of the problem – the respiratory tract and lungs – without having to go through the bloodstream, as happens with pills or syrups. Because of this:

- you get more rapid, targeted results
- a lower dose can be prescribed

- there is less risk of side-effects, which is particularly important if your child is taking steroids.

So it is well worth persevering with inhaled medication, even if you have a few hiccups to start with.

Very young children, however, are often prescribed reliever drugs (salbutamol and terbutaline) in syrup form, taken on a regular basis like preventers, because they cannot manage the inhaled method. Taking the drugs in this form means they have to go through the bloodstream to get to the lungs, rather than going straight to the trouble spot, which has two effects: they do not work as quickly as inhaled medication and they have to be given at a much higher dose, which in turn increases the risk of side effects. All these reasons mean your doctor will encourage your child to move onto inhaled medication as soon as she is able.

In acute episodes of asthma, when an attack needs to be brought under control quickly, your child may be prescribed a course of prednisolone, a corticosteroid which comes in tablet, soluble or syrup form for very young children. It is an emergency rescue treatment, taken until the attack stabilizes and the symptoms die down. Prednisolone may also be prescribed in cases of severe asthma which cannot be controlled using inhaled preventers alone. But it would only be prescribed for children if absolutely necessary, and your doctor would stop or reduce the dose as soon as symptoms allowed.

Getting into a routine
It can be easy to forget to give your child her daily preventers if she has no asthma symptoms. But to keep the condition away, these drugs need to be taken whether there are symptoms or not. So it is a good idea to get into a routine. With inhaled steroids, which usually have to be taken twice a day, it is easy to establish a routine, taking them in the morning and last thing at night. Learning to associate it with another regular activity, like brushing your teeth, helps. With sodium cromoglycate, which has to be taken up to four times daily, it is slightly more difficult, although it is logical to get into the habit of taking it around mealtimes (breakfast, lunch, tea) and then before bed.

Reliever medication is only taken when it is needed, but should always be carried with you. If possible, have two canisters on the go: one for your bag or pocket and one for home. Schoolchildren will have to take one to school with them, either keeping it themselves in a schoolbag or giving it to a teacher or the school nurse. (For more on managing at school, *see* chapter 6.)

ARE THERE ANY SIDE-EFFECTS?

There are not many drugs which do not have side-effects and asthma treatments are no exception, although progress in refining both the drugs and the method of delivery have meant that adverse reactions can be kept to a minimum. Whether your child will suffer any side-effects depends on her individual susceptibility and how much medication she is taking. Bronchodilators have been associated with side-effects like increased heart rate, trembling and headaches, and several studies have also raised concerns that overuse of relievers can make asthma symptoms worse.

But the biggest worry for parents is that their child is on steroids from a very young age, and used orally over a long period, they have an alarmingly long list of possible side-effects, from skin thinning and lowered immunity to growth retardation, diabetes, glaucoma and osteoporosis. High doses for extended periods may also affect the functioning of the adrenal glands. Steroids are actually synthetic versions of the hormone cortisone, which is produced naturally in the body by the adrenal glands, which lie just above the kidneys. If you constantly put high levels of synthetic cortisone into the system, these glands stop producing the hormone (called adrenal suppression). If steroid treatment is then suddenly withdrawn it can cause metabolic breakdown in the body. If your child is on long-term steroid tablets, she should carry an asthma card stating as much in case of accident. Hospital staff will need to give her additional steroids to prompt the recovery process.

These possible side-effects can be worrying, but you have to place them in the context of your child's asthma. Asthma is a serious condition which can be debilitating if untreated, stopping a child from living a carefree, normal life. It can also be fatal. Moreover, around 80 per cent of children with asthma have it mildly to moderately. This means it can usually be controlled with low-dose inhaled steroids, which have a very low risk of side-effects. Occasional courses of steroid tablets or syrup to bring an asthma attack under control have also been shown to carry little long-term risk.

The greatest risk is for those children with more severe asthma, who need high-dose inhaled steroids and frequent or prolonged courses of oral steroids. These children are carefully monitored by their doctors, who will make regular checks on growth rate, weight and general development. They should review the treatment every three to six months with a view to decreasing the dose of medication where possible. And with regard to adrenal suppression, doctors do not simply stop steroid treatment if a patient has been on high doses for a prolonged period. Patients are gradually weaned off treatment, allowing the adrenal glands to normalize their production of natural cortisone.

Complementary therapies can help in keeping your child's medication needs as low as possible; some children have even been able to come off conventional medication with regular complementary treatment. Parents, too, have an important role to play. You know your child best and may notice changes which your doctor could miss. Signs that steroid treatment is causing problems include repeated viral and other infections, which indicate that her immune system is not working up to par, bruising easily, tiredness and listlessness, and an increase in weight.

If you are at all worried, talk to your doctor, tell her what you have noted and point out your worries. If steroid treatment is causing side-effects, you and your doctor will need to reassess the treatment programme, weighing up the risks of treatment against the benefits, and perhaps trying to lower the dosage being taken or moving to different medication.

You can also help cut down on the risk of side-effects in other ways.

• Make sure your child eats a healthy, balanced diet, packed with immune-boosting nutrients (*see* chapter 2).

- Check that she is using her preventer inhaler correctly, so lessening the chances of an attack and the need for a course of steroid tablets.
- Do not let her overuse reliever drugs. Always believe her if she says she needs her inhaler, but try to teach her to use it judiciously.
- See a complementary therapist who can help get your child into a state of good general health to fight both the symptoms of asthma and the effects of drug treatment (*see* chapter 5).

Possible side-effects

Whether your child will suffer side-effects from asthma treatments depends on her age and susceptibility, so the threshold dosages given below are only approximate.

- *Sodium cromoglycate*. May cause coughing after breathing in
- *Inhaled corticosteroids*. Low doses (less than 800 mcg daily): hoarseness; oral candidiasis (thrush), although washing your child's mouth out after inhaling can help avoid this; higher doses (over 1 mg daily): skin thinning, easy bruising, lowered immunity to infection, stunted growth
- *Corticosteroid tablets/syrups (prednisolone)*. If used long-term: osteoporosis (thinning of the bones), diabetes, cataracts, glaucoma, muscle weakness and wasting, water retention, weight gain, Cushing's syndrome (characterized by a moon face, high blood pressure, hump on the back of the neck and muscle weakness), adrenal suppression
- *Long-acting beta2-agonists*. Accelerated heart rate, abnormal heartbeat, anxiety, muscle tremors, headache; fewer side-effects are experienced with inhaled medication compared to tablets/syrup

Relievers

- *Short-acting beta2-agonists*. Accelerated heart rate, abnormal heartbeat, muscle tremors, headache, anxiety/irritability, hyperactivity; fewer side effects are experienced with inhaled medication compared to tablets/syrup
- *Theophylline*. Nausea and vomiting, and if levels become too concentrated in the blood, abnormal heartbeat and seizures; it is usually given only in low doses and any child taking it should have her blood levels checked regularly

WHAT TO DO IN AN ATTACK

Both you and your doctor will aim to avoid an asthma attack, and it is hoped that with treatment, monitoring and trigger-avoidance tactics, emergencies will be rare. But a lot depends on how serious your child's asthma is. Severe cases are more likely to break through the protective cover of preventive treatment and these children need very careful monitoring. It also depends on the triggers which set your child's asthma off. Certain times of year – for example, the pollen season or as it gets colder – may make some children's asthma harder to control, and parents need to be prepared for this. The most common trigger of all is a cold – few children escape without two or three colds in a year – so it is always wise to look out for a worsening of symptoms around an infection.

What is important is that you and your child:

- know the triggers which exacerbate her symptoms
- monitor asthma on a day-to-day basis to ensure that the symptoms are not deteriorating
- recognize the signs of an imminent attack
- have a management plan to get the asthma under control again (*see* chapter 1).

Recognizing the signs

An attack may be on the horizon if:

- symptoms deteriorate or develop, ie coughing (especially at night), wheezing, breathing difficulties
- unusual symptoms develop – eg lightheadedness, nausea or itchiness – which many parents learn to recognize as a warning signal in their child
- in children who can give peak flow readings, the peak expiratory flow falls and/or there are unusual dips in PEF in the morning
- your child is using her reliever more than usual, or the effect is not lasting four hours

Making an emergency spacer
If your child's symptoms worsen while you are away from home and you do not have your spacer with you, you can make an emergency spacer from a paper or a plastic cup. Simply make a hole in the bottom and push the inhaler mouth through it. Place the cup over your child's mouth and tell her to breathe in steadily and regularly. Once a breathing pattern is established, 'puff' the inhaler into the cup. Keep it there for several breaths.

Your next step depends on your child and her asthma picture; if you have a management plan, this should tell you what to do at this stage. It may, however, go something like this:

Give your child extra relieving treatment. If the symptoms then subside, the relieving treatment lasts for four hours or more and PEF improves (to 80 per cent or more of your child's normal best reading), you have warded off the attack. Always contact your doctor for follow-up advice. If, after giving extra relieving treatment, the symptoms improve but do not go away completely, or if they subside but return in less than four hours, seek medical advice urgently.

If, after extra relieving treatment, there is no difference in symptoms or they get worse, or if the PEF is dropping, take your child to a hospital emergency department or call an ambulance. Make sure that you arrange for the ambulance to carry oxygen and a nebulizer. In the meantime, keep giving your child her reliever through a spacer every two to five minutes. (There is no danger of overdosing.) If you have an emergency course of steroid tablets with you, start giving them as soon as the symptoms start to deteriorate, and inform your doctor or the hospital that you have started the course.

Finally, in an emergency, try to stay calm – your child will not be helped by seeing you panicking and it may add to her own distress. Do not be afraid to skip steps on the management plan, either, if you feel the situation is acute. It is always better to be safe than sorry.

SIGNS OF AN EMERGENCY
- normal relieving treatment has no effect on symptoms
- your child cannot talk
- breathing is severely laboured
- pulse is rapid (over 140 beats per minute in a child)
- her face is pale, with blue tinge
- she is very drowsy or lethargic and seems confused
- wheezing stops (so-called 'silent chest')

If your child shows any of these symptoms, get medical assistance urgently; call an ambulance and say you will need oxygen and a nebulizer, or take your child to a hospital emergency department yourself.

Hospital stays

These days, stays in hospital are usually short, and only last until the attack has been brought under control and the doctors can see the child is making good progress. Hospitals can, however, be frightening and distressing for a child, so make it easier for her.

- Prepare her beforehand, when she is not in the middle of an attack. Read books about going to hospital – there are some very good ones aimed at young children. Explain what will happen at the accident and emergency unit, who the doctors and nurses are and what they do. Your child will probably be put on a nebulizer; if she has not used one before, explain to her what one is and show pictures.
- If you have other children, have a stand-by babysitter ready to come over in an emergency to look after them, so that you do not have to worry about brothers and sisters as well as the child with asthma.
- If possible, stay with her in the emergency ward, even if you just remain discreetly in the background as the medical staff get the attack under control.
- If an overnight stay is needed, stay with your child; most hospitals will now arrange for a cot bed to be set up.
- Bring, or arrange to be brought in, nightclothes, toothbrushes,

towel, teddies and toys. Bringing a little bit of home into the hospital can make it seem less austere.

- If you cannot stay during the day, visit whenever you can, even if she cries when you go. Most children will cry, but they would feel even more abandoned if you stayed away in case they became upset.
- Be extra loving at a time when she will be feeling a little lost and worried about what has happened. Doctors and nurses will undoubtedly be friendly and reassuring, but it is your words which count.

Chapter Five

Complementary Approaches

More and more people are discovering how much complementary therapies like homeopathy, acupuncture and osteopathy can help overcome or improve seemingly intractable health problems. In a recent survey of Consumers' Association members in the UK, around a third had seen a complementary practitioner for a health problem; of these, 83 per cent said they felt better afterwards. An American survey found that around a third of adults had used complementary therapies while a 1996 Australian study established that one in five of the population regularly visited a complementary practitioner. Moreover, an increasing number of conventional health professionals accept that complementary approaches have a role to play in health care. A UK government survey found that 40 per cent of doctors in England offered patients some kind of complementary therapy.

Complementary therapies can be effective in cases of asthma, particularly in children, because they often respond better and more quickly than adults since problems tend not to be so deep-rooted – so you could see results quite rapidly. They can help in the following ways, depending on which therapy you choose:

- They are concerned with 'whole-body' health, which means they do not concentrate solely on your child's asthma but work towards building up his health and immunity generally. In this way, he will be stronger and fitter, and his immune system will be better able to fight off the effects of pollution, allergens, infections and so on.

- They can alleviate inflammation and muscle spasm, even though the approaches to doing so may differ considerably.
- They can relieve stress and anxiety and help your child to relax.
- They can promote better breathing habits.
- Because they focus as much on the emotional and spiritual elements of illness as on the physical, they can ease cases of asthma which have an emotional trigger as well as helping your child cope better with his condition.

With asthma the aim of complementary therapy is not to take over from conventional treatments, but to alleviate symptoms alongside them. Both your doctor and your complementary therapist will be working towards keeping your child's need for medication at as low a dose as possible. In milder cases, regular complementary health care may be all that is needed to keep asthma away.

Case Study

'Sean developed asthma at four and a half,' says Siobhan. 'He started off on a bronchodilator but moved on to sodium cromoglycate through an inhaler after a few months, coupled with occasional puffs of his reliever. He was fine with this for around a year but then we moved house and his asthma just went haywire. On two occasions, we rushed him to hospital because the medication didn't seem to be making any difference. He changed to inhaled steroids but he still kept having to take courses of steroid tablets to keep the asthma in check. Then someone at my eldest son's school mentioned that her son's asthma had been helped with acupuncture, and she gave me the phone number of her acupuncturist.

'I hadn't had much to do with alternative therapies before this, so it was a big step for me to take, but you get so desperate to find something that will help. Anyway, I've no regrets. Although improvements weren't dramatic, over the past year we've gradually lowered his dose of preventer and have recently been able to drop it altogether. Sean now just takes the reliever when he gets wheezy, usually when he exercises or if the weather is really cold.'

It is important, when you start seeing a complementary therapist, that you do not suddenly stop taking conventional medication in favour of a wholly alternative approach. Ideally, you should inform your doctor that you are seeing a complementary therapist so that they can work together to alleviate your child's asthma. In practice, this may not be possible; although more doctors are accepting complementary therapies, they are often reluctant to work with them or do not know enough about the approaches to get involved. If your doctor is not open to complementary approaches, keep your therapist informed of what medication your child is on and make sure you continue to attend regular assessments with your doctor or at the asthma clinic. If all goes well, you will begin to see an improvement in your child's symptoms, with a corresponding drop in his need for medication.

It is also inadvisable to treat your child yourself with over-the-counter preparations such as supplements or herbal tablets. This can be a temptation, particularly with vitamin or mineral supplements; you may hear about something being good for asthma and start dosing your child in the hope that it will help. But asthma is such an individual condition, with triggers, severity and frequency of episodes varying from child to child and from one attack to another. It is a condition which needs individual assessment and specially tailored treatment; self-treating your child may miss the mark completely and therefore be a waste of money. You are far better off spending your money on seeing a well-qualified and experienced complementary practitioner who will give your child an in-depth assessment and offer treatment accordingly.

Once complementary treatment is under way, watch your child for signs that asthma symptoms are getting worse and inform your therapist of any changes. With complementary treatments, patients often go through an acute stage, where symptoms do get worse, but this should only last a short while (one or two days in most cases) and then your child should start making progress. This acute stage is not the time to give up on complementary treatment – it is actually a sign that it is working. However, if symptoms get worse and continue that way, talk over your options with your therapist, but do not feel you have to carry on if you are not happy it is helping. With any form of treatment – conventional or complementary – you should try it, but if it is not helping do not carry on with it.

Choosing a therapist

Asthma is a serious condition, and it is extremely important that you feel confident the therapist you are seeing is properly qualified. The field of alternative health care is largely unregulated, although most therapies now have some kind of regulatory body which sets standards of training and qualifications, provides insurance and ensures that members work to a code of ethics. These bodies can provide members of the public with a register of practitioners who practise to their standard. You will find them listed in the 'Useful Addresses' section at the end of the book. There are a number of steps you can take to ensure your child receives quality complementary health care.

- If your doctor is open to complementary approaches, ask if he can recommend a local practitioner whom he has worked with before. Failing this, try the asthma nurse, who may have more contact with asthma patients who have tried complementary therapies. Another approach is to find someone you know who can recommend an alternative practitioner.
- If you have decided to try a complementary approach but do not have any 'leads', you can start looking in one of two ways: either decide which therapy you would like to try, approach the self-regulating body for that therapy and ask for their register of practitioners. You could also ask if any of their members specialize in treating children or asthma. Alternatively, you can look through the local telephone directory. Approach two or three therapists and check their qualifications, training and fees before deciding. Ensure that the practitioner is a member of the self-regulating body for his therapy; phone the relevant organization to ensure that he is on their register, do not take his word for it.
- Think about the therapy itself: is your child likely to be comfortable with it? Therapies vary a lot in their approach, as you will see from the descriptions given briefly below. Your child may be happier with some approaches than others. If, for example, he is not one for cuddling or physical touch, avoid therapies like osteopathy or massage; if you have difficulty

getting your child to take medicine, herbs may present problems – fresh herbal mixtures can taste pretty vile! Also, some therapies call for a different mind-set to conventional thinking – for example, the traditional Chinese approach involving yin and yang forces and energy pathways through the body. This may be unsettling for a teenager used to the Western approach to health and disease, although a younger child will not be bothered by the philosophy behind treatment.

- Do you and your child feel comfortable with the practitioner? He may be fully qualified and experienced in treating asthma, but if you do not get on then the treatment may well be affected. Remember that the complementary approach usually means longer appointments and a lot more talking than we are used to in conventional practice; you need to feel at ease with the person you are opening up to.
- Be wary of any practitioner who wants your child to stop his regular medication. A proficient therapist can work with conventional treatments until a point is reached when dosage can be gradually and safely lowered.

WHICH THERAPY?

There are a vast number of therapies on offer now and the choice can be confusing. A lot comes down to which approach your child feels most comfortable with. Generally, the therapies outlined in this book fall into a number of categories, with some overlaps: manipulative (osteopathy), postural (Alexander technique, yoga), medicinal (homeopathy, herbalism), psychological (hypnotherapy, autogenic training), touch (massage, reflexology) and practical self-help (Alexander technique, yoga, relaxation). The descriptions below will give you an idea of what is involved in each therapy.

Where you live also plays a part. If you do not want to travel a long way for each appointment, then you will have to choose a local practitioner. The chances are you will find a practitioner in your area for one of the more well-known therapies – acupuncture, homeopathy, osteopathy – but not for less well-known therapies like autogenic training or the Buteyko method.

I have focused on therapies which have a track record in

helping with asthma, either because they are well established and research studies have shown they can help, or because there is a substantial amount of positive anecdotal evidence. But the list is by no means exhaustive, and you may know of practitioners in therapies not covered here who have had success with asthma.

Acupuncture and traditional Chinese medicine (TCM)

Although acupuncture has only become established in the West over the past 20–30 years, it has been used for many thousands of years in the East to treat a wide range of complaints. Acupuncture is actually part of a whole system of traditional Chinese medicine which includes herbals, diet, massage and gentle exercises called qi gong. In the West, however, acupuncture is often used on its own and many conventional health professionals – doctors, midwives and nurses – have learnt the techniques.

The philosophy behind TCM is very different from the Western view of health; according to Chinese belief, the key to health lies in balance (yin and yang). There is balance in everything in the universe: left and right, man and woman, hot and cold, hard and soft, and so on. The same is true when it comes to good health: when there is balance in the body, we are healthy. Healthy balance relies on the smooth flow of a vital life-giving energy called qi (pronounced 'chee') through channels or meridians in the body. Imbalances occur when there are blockages or weaknesses in the flow of this energy, or if outside influences like excessive heat, cold or damp get into the body.

Acupuncture involves using very fine needles, inserted at strategic points (acupoints) in the body, to stimulate the flow of vital energy and correct imbalances.

When it comes to asthma, an acupuncturist or doctor of Chinese medicine assesses each case individually. In TCM diagnosis, signs and symptoms may indicate a problem with the lungs, but it could also be kidney imbalance, as well as outside influences like damp and cold. Your acupuncturist will reach a diagnosis by taking your child's pulses (according to TCM, there are three on each wrist), looking at his tongue and complexion, listening to him cough and breathe, and taking down details of his medical history, lifestyle, sleep patterns, eating habits, likes and dislikes, and so on. From this, he will decide on treatment, often using a combination of acupuncture, herbs and moxibustion (where herbs are burnt over an acupoint without touching the skin).

Parents often worry that acupuncture will hurt, but all your child should feel is a pinprick as the needles are inserted and then sometimes a tingling sensation or numbness around the insertion point. The needles are usually left in for around 20 minutes. Your child may feel a little sleepy after treatment, but this is normal.

Acupuncture without needles
It may be difficult to persuade your child that acupuncture needles will not hurt (it can be difficult to persuade many adults!), but there is now an alternative in *laser acupuncture*, which is often used on children. Nothing breaks the skin; a small pen-like instrument is simply held on the spot, and a low-dose laser beam stimulates the acupoint. Your child will feel nothing.

Also becoming more popular is *ultrasound acupuncture*, which works in the same way, while *acupressure*, where the therapist applies pressure to the acupoints in place of needles, can also be very effective for children.

Alexander technique

An Alexander practitioner is not a therapist but a teacher; your child will learn how to change his postural behaviour and use his body more efficiently, which may mean unlearning bad posture habits and re-establishing his natural balance and mobility. The Alexander technique has a good background in helping with breathing disorders, including asthma, because it allows you to lengthen your body, open out your chest and generally establish better freedom of movement. Many singers and actors swear by it as a means of keeping them in good voice. It also teaches you how to let go of body tension and mental stress, another aspect of the technique which can help those with asthma.

It takes around 30 lessons to learn the technique and then your child should be able to build the postural changes and simple exercises into his life so that they become second nature. The additional benefits are good posture, a confident bearing and a relaxed, tension-free body – something most parents would like for their child, whether they have asthma or not!

Autogenic training (AT)

AT is another therapy where you are more of a pupil than a patient. It is basically a form of deep relaxation; through a series of mental exercises, you are taught to influence your autonomic nervous system so that it does not respond to stress but, in stressful situations, switches on your relaxation response instead. For this reason, it is often useful for stress-triggered asthma; several studies have also shown that it can be of benefit psychologically in that it helps someone with asthma feel more in control. AT is taught over eight to ten weeks, and you should practise for 15 minutes, three times a day. It is unsuitable for young children, but teenagers may find that it helps them deal better with stress while helping to control the symptoms.

Bio-resonance therapy

This newish therapy uses a machine to measure the electromagnetic frequencies emitted by the body; strong waves indicate all is well, while weak or fluctuating waves indicate a problem. This information can then be used to treat allergies and intolerances. The therapist will place a phial of a suspected allergen either in the machine or on your child's body, and will then measure the degree of sensitivity registered in the body's electromagnetic responses. Once an allergen is tracked down, the machine can turn the disrupted waves around and reflect them back into the body, rebalancing it so it no longer responds to the allergen. It is safe for children, who often respond to treatment very quickly.

Herbal medicine

This is often also called medical herbalism or Western herbalism to distinguish it from Chinese or Indian (Ayurvedic) herbalism, although they all have much in common. European herbalism has a long history behind it, with folk remedies handed down from generation to generation until the great herbalists of the 16th and 17th centuries – Paracelsus, Nicholas Culpeper and William Turner – produced herbal remedy books based on their own medical experiences. Many modern drugs come from herbs: aspirin from willow bark, morphine from poppies, atropine from deadly nightshade and the antispasmodic ephedrine – which is sometimes used in asthma treatment – from *Ephedra sinica* (also known as *ma huang*).

There are a number of herbs which can help with asthma, including *Ephedra sinica*, Roman chamomile, which has an antispasmodic, anti-inflammatory effect, and eucalyptus, another antispasmodic and expectorant. The remedies come in the form of tinctures, essential oils, infusions or decoctions, where you boil up the leaves, flowers, roots or bark yourself to create a tea (*see* box below).

You may be worried about the dangers of giving a child herbal preparations – herbs are potent medicines, which is why they have such a therapeutic effect when used by a qualified therapist. But they are quite safe as long as you see a qualified medical herbalist and keep him informed of what prescription medication your child is taking.

Making up herbal treatments
A herbalist may prescribe a herbal remedy to be taken in a number of ways.
- **As a tincture.** This is made by steeping dried or fresh herbs in a mixture of alcohol and water. It is taken diluted in water or, for children, it can be made less bitter by mixing it with fruit juice.
- **As an essential oil.** The oil is extracted from the plant and bottled. Essential oils in herbal medicine are used as steam inhalants, in chest rubs and for massage, when they are mixed with a carrier oil.

- **As an infusion**. Dried or fresh flowers and leaves are steeped in hot, freshly boiled water and left to infuse for 10–15 minutes. The strained 'tea' is then drunk, one cupful three times a day.
- **As a decoction**. This method is used for roots, bark and twigs. Herbs are brought to the boil in water and allowed to simmer for an hour. The strained tea is drunk as for an infusion.

Some herbal remedies, particularly in Chinese herbalism, also come in tablets.

Homeopathy

Often paraphrased as 'treating like with like', the basis of homeo-pathic treatment is that you can cure an illness by treating it with minute doses of a substance which – in larger doses – would cause symptoms similar to the illness. The remedies themselves contain such diluted quantities of the original active ingredient that it cannot even be picked up in tests, yet homeopaths have found that the more diluted the remedy is, the stronger the effect it has. Remedies come as small white pills, powders or liquid and are completely tasteless, so they are not difficult to get a child to take. You simply place a pill under the tongue and let it dissolve. How many you take, and how often, depends on the symptoms.

With asthma, a homeopath will first give your child remedies to get the acute symptoms under control. But the long-term aim is to treat him constitutionally, which means finding a particular remedy suited to his personality, susceptibilities and general characteristics. This remedy should work to keep his whole body and mind in a state of healthy balance. To establish your child's constitutional type, a homeopath will ask a lot of questions at your first appointment which may seem unrelated to health or asthma, like what time of day your child likes best, his favourite foods, or whether he prefers hot or cold weather. The answers will help the homeopath build up a remedy picture of him and decide which remedy to offer.

Homeopathy is completely safe and particularly suited to children, who often respond very quickly to the remedies.

Case Study

'After seeing my homeopath for a number of months and being impressed that she was able to help with my problems, I mentioned about bringing Doug along,' says Jackie about her six-year-old asthmatic son. 'He suffers from allergic asthma, which is triggered by dust and pollens. My homeopath felt she would be able to help his asthma, so we started treatment. At first, he seemed to get worse and he was having to use his reliever more than usual, but I stuck to it despite a few worries. But this stage only lasted a day or two and then, quite rapidly, the symptoms dried up. Apparently, symptoms often do get worse before they get better. At our next appointment, Doug was given a different remedy and there was no looking back. Doug still has a problem around pollen time, but he doesn't suffer the chronic symptoms he used to and I make sure I take him for a homeopathic booster just before the pollen season begins.'

Hypnotherapy

Hypnotherapy is a form of deep relaxation, where the patient is helped into a trance-like state by a therapist, who then makes suggestions for changes in his thinking and beliefs about illness. What hypnotherapy is *not* is showtime hypnosis, where a hypnotist appears to make people do things against their will. Your child is always in control and can choose to pick up a suggestion or not. This is probably why some people find hypnotherapy effective and others do not when, for example, trying to stop smoking. You have to be highly motivated to want to do what the therapist is suggesting if your thinking is going to change.

That said, children usually react well to hypnotherapy, because they have less entrenched perceptions about change and are highly motivated to improve their symptoms. It has been shown to give good results in helping with stress-induced asthma and in lessening the tension and panic which exacerbate an asthma attack. An added bonus of hypnotherapy is that your child can be taught self-hypnosis techniques to draw on in times of stress and tension, and studies have found that self-hypnosis can significantly help children with asthma. In addition, a form of hypnotherapy called hypnohealing has had some success: the patient is encouraged to think positive about his illness, imagining healthy cells fighting the allergen, inflammation going down, airways opening, and so on. It is being used more and more in cancer therapy, and gut-directed hypnotherapy, which utilizes similar techniques, is a well-established approach to controlling irritable bowel.

Therapies for stress
In addition to the therapies mentioned here, other approaches to stress relief and relaxation include:

- **Aromatherapy.**   This therapy utilizes the healing properties of plant oils, either using them, mixed with a carrier oil, in massage or burning them in burners or vaporizers. Good oils for beating stress include: lavender, clary sage, neroli, jasmine, bergamot and sandalwood.
- **Flower remedies.**   These are aimed purely at helping emotional problems and many people swear by them. You will find a range of remedies available, including American, Australian, South African and Bach remedies. With Bach remedies, try vervain for stress, rock water or impatiens if you find it difficult to relax, and vervain, rock water or vine for tension.
- **Massage therapy.**   There are many different types of massage, the most commonly available in the West being traditional Swedish massage, which has a good track record in relieving tension and helping you relax. It involves a variety of strokes which smooth away areas of tension while stimulating muscles and circulation.
- **Meditation.**   The main forms of meditation in the West are Buddhist and Transcendental, both of which relax, induce calmness and lower stress levels and general agitation.
- **T'ai chi.**   These gentle movements form part of traditional Chinese therapy and are actually a form of kung fu – a non-violent martial art. The slow, gentle movements are excellent for calming, destressing and focusing the mind.

Naturopathy

This therapy originated in the 19th century and is based on maximizing the healing properties in nature. It involves nutritional advice, water therapy, relaxation and stress management, osteopathy and sometimes colonic cleansing, and many naturopaths now also incorporate homeopathy or herbs into their therapy. Although it is primarily involved in boosting the immune system, it can also help in cases of asthma by reducing inflammation, stimulating circulation, helping with stress, tracking down food allergies or intolerances and relieving any muscular tension. In experienced hands, naturopathy is quite safe for children.

Nutritional therapy

There is a growing bank of evidence to show that bad diet increases the risk of developing a plethora of modern-day ills, from diabetes and heart disease to infertility and cancer. Nutritional therapy takes this one step further by using nutrients therapeutically to overcome illness. You could say that in nutritional therapy, vitamins, minerals and other nutrients become our medicines.

With asthma, a nutritional therapist will first assess your child's diet and nutritional status to ensure that his symptoms are not caused by deficiencies. He will also look for signs of a toxic overload from food sources (agrochemicals, additives, preservatives and other contaminants) and inhaled pollutants, which could exacerbate the asthma as well as depleting nutrients in the body. Lastly, he will investigate whether your child's asthma is caused by a food intolerance.

Each asthma case is unique, in nutritional terms as in all others, and is affected by current diet, toxicity levels, allergies or intolerances, nutritional deficiencies and what foods your child likes or dislikes. The therapist will also want to know about any other niggling problems like headaches, rashes or tiredness, which may seem unconnected with the asthma but which could indicate a deficiency. If he suspects that a food intolerance is at the root of your child's asthma, he may put him on an elimination diet or run allergen tests to see if any foods prompt an allergic reaction.

Nutritional therapy is very safe in qualified hands, as the

therapist will ensure that your child is getting all the nutrients he needs for a healthy diet and that any supplementation is within safe limits. Diet plans are flexible, adapting easily to a child's age and needs, and may even encourage your child to eat a healthier diet. (For more on diet and food intolerances generally, *see* chapter 2).

Osteopathy

Probably now the most 'mainstream' complementary therapy, osteopathy is concerned with restoring balance to the body's structure (skeleton, joints, muscles, ligaments and connective tissue) when it has been thrown out by injuries and strain, poor posture, or the effects of emotional upheaval. Although it is best known for helping with more structurally related problems, like a bad back or slipped disc, osteopathy can also help with asthma. It eases muscular tension and, of course, muscular spasm of the airways is one of the precipitating factors in an asthma attack. Its techniques also relax muscles generally and an osteopath will focus on areas of muscular tension in the throat and around the ribs and diaphragm, as well as getting the lymphatic system working efficiently so that excess fluids are cleared out of the system more quickly – important in asthma when there is a build-up of mucus.

Osteopathy is not painful and is safe for children; some osteopaths specialize in treating children and may call themselves paediatric osteopaths.

Reflexology

Another 'energy' therapy similar to traditional Chinese medicine and acupuncture, reflexology is said to work by clearing blockages in the flow of vital energy around the body and stimulating organs. Unlike acupuncture, it does not do this via acupoints but by the gentle massage of 'reflex zones' on the feet and hands.

The body is divided into ten zones: imagine a line going

vertically down the centre of your body with five zones on each side of that line. Blockages along a zone line will affect any part of the body that rests within that zone. The zones end at your feet and at your hands, where there are points mirroring all the different parts of the body – organs, bones, glands and so on. For every point on the feet, there is a corresponding one on the hands, so reflexology can be performed on either to get the same effect, although reflexologists prefer to work with the feet.

Of particular interest in asthma are the reflex points for the lungs and chest, which lie in the middle of the soft padded area just below the toes. On the hands, the corresponding points are located in the middle of the fleshy pad just below the fingers. The reflexologist would look for crystals in these areas – slight swellings or lumps which indicate a blockage. By gently but firmly working the area with his fingers, he can break down the crystals and clear the blockage, getting energy flowing along the zone line again and correcting any symptoms caused by the blockage.

Reflexology has been shown to improve the symptoms of asthma and can help with stress, as it is one of the most relaxing of therapies. Most children enjoy having their feet massaged, although young children are usually given a shorter session with gentler strokes, as they do not need as much stimulation as adults.

Yoga

Most people are familiar with yoga as a form of exercise, but from ancient times it has been practised in the East as a way of maximizing and maintaining health. There are different styles of yoga, the most common in the West being Hatha or Iyengar yoga, but each involves the same basic format: stretching exercises or postures, breathing practice and meditation.

As well as improving general health and fitness, studies show that yoga can be of considerable help to people with asthma and other respiratory disorders. The breathing exercises are particularly useful in stopping asthma sufferers falling into the habit of shallow breathing. Both postures and breathing can strengthen the lungs and improve the circulation as more oxygen is getting into the body. The meditational side of yoga will also help your child relax and let go of tension, which should in turn ease the symptoms of asthma and help him cope better in an attack.

Case Study

'I really believe yoga has helped me,' says ten-year-old Nicola. 'I feel very good after a class – my body is loose and relaxed. A lot of my asthma stems from worry and yoga has also helped me to cope with that. When I find myself getting worked up about something, I stop, think about relaxing and calm myself down. I've started to learn the clarinet now and I think yoga breathing is helping me there, too.'

Yoga is very child-friendly and you may be lucky enough to find a children's class running in your area. The movements are slow and gentle and your child will only be encouraged to do what he feels able to, although to get full benefit, he should practise every day, building it into his life. Always inform the yoga teacher that your child has asthma.

Could asthma be caused by overbreathing?

A new approach to controlling asthma is through the Buteyko method, a series of lessons in which people are taught specific breathing techniques. The method hails from Russia, where physiologist Professor Konstantin Buteyko undertook research into breathing and health and discovered a link between overbreathing and respiratory illnesses; he found that asthmatics in particular breathed three or more times over the recommended 'normal' level. By teaching people with asthma to breathe normally, Buteyko found their symptoms could be radically improved and their reliance on drug treatment lessened.

Buteyko practitioners believe overbreathing can cause asthma because it depletes the lungs' store of carbon dioxide, which is needed in the right ratio to release oxygen into the bloodstream. If the lungs' stock of carbon dioxide runs too low, the lungs shut down in protest: airways constrict, inflammation results and the symptoms of asthma develop.

The Buteyko method marks a radical departure in thinking

about the causes of asthma and is the subject of considerable controversy, particularly since practitioners claim a 90 per cent success rate (success being judged as needing less or no medication). In Russia, several trials have shown that it can help asthmatics and it was approved by the Russian Ministry of Health in the 1980s. In the West, a controlled trial at Queensland University in Australia found that patients with asthma reduced their use of relieving medication by 90 per cent.

Patients learn the breathing techniques over a short course of one-hour sessions, either in a group or one to one. The course focuses first on using the techniques to overcome an asthma attack before moving on to retrain the brain to breathe correctly through a series of exercises. Currently, however, there are very few teachers of the method in the West and the course is expensive.

Chapter Six

As They Grow

Although there are many steps parents can take generally to help a child with asthma, some of the advice changes or has more relevance at particular times. You will have to take responsibility for making sure your baby or toddler takes her medication, for example, but at some point you will also have to hand that responsibility over to her. As children grow up, new challenges arise: school is the greatest step from the age of five, as they learn to manage their condition outside the home environment. For teenagers, there are the stresses of becoming an adult – examination pressure, thinking about a career, becoming more independent and eventually moving away from home.

THE PRESCHOOL YEARS: FROM BIRTH TO FIVE

The is probably the most difficult time for parents with an asthmatic child. First, it can be hard to have asthma conventionally diagnosed at a very young age and so get speedy treatment (although complementary treatment – which does not deal so much in symptoms but in the total picture – should be able to help if your doctor cannot). Secondly, you have to take responsibility for monitoring and controlling your child's asthma while she is too young in many cases to tell you how she feels. However, there are plenty of positive steps you can take to ensure that asthma does not get in the way of your child enjoying the preschool years with you.

Feeding in the first year

The general dietary guidelines given in chapter 2 for all children are also applicable to those under five. However, there are a few additional suggestions for the early years, specifically to do with weaning and dealing with fussy toddler eaters. It appears that a baby's diet in the early months is an important indicator of whether she will develop an allergic-related condition or not. If there is a history of asthma or allergy-related conditions, keeping to these guidelines may offer your child some protection.

- Breastfeed for at least the first six months. This certainly seems to provide some protection against allergic conditions of this type. Formula milk has improved immensely over the years, but there are components of breast milk that formula manufacturers cannot replicate, particularly the protective antibodies which come through from the mother in the first days after the birth. If there is a strong family history of food allergy, it may also be worthwhile avoiding common allergy-causing foods while breastfeeding, as what the mother eats and drinks goes through to the milk.

  If you are having problems getting breastfeeding to go smoothly, do not give up; get in touch with a breastfeeding organization like La Lèche League, who have a network of local breastfeeding counsellors on hand to help you to overcome any initial difficulties and get you into a routine of breastfeeding comfortably. Once you are up and away, there is usually no looking back.

- Do not introduce solids too early. Sometimes parents feel under pressure to introduce solids as early as possible, but if your baby may be susceptible to asthma it is worth keeping to a wholly milk diet for the first six months to offer her maximum protection. Breast milk is a complete food which adapts to your baby's nutritional needs and there is no pressing need to introduce solids before the six-month mark. If you do start weaning before this time, do not begin earlier than four months and offer only very bland purées – baby rice, apple, pear, banana – and slowly introduce a wider variety, one food at a time. Avoid common allergy-causing foods and certainly do not introduce gluten (anything containing wheat like cereals and biscuits) before six months. Look out for gluten-free baby foods; there are gluten-free products (breads, biscuits, etc) available from health food stores and chemists. If you are particularly worried about food allergies (for instance, if you, your partner or a close family member suffers from the problem), talk to your health practitioner about your baby's diet.

- Leave introducing cow's milk until one year old. In a family with a history of allergy, stick with breast milk or formula, coupled with a steadily increasing solid-food diet, for the first year before introducing plain cow's milk, as this is strongly associated with triggering an allergic reaction. Just one bottle may be enough. You can use expressed breast milk or formula for mixing up cereals and other foods. Dairy products like cheese and yoghurt can be introduced before this, once your baby is eating a good mixture of other foods.

Dealing with fussy eaters

After weaning, the toddler years are often a time of dietary despair for parents, who are thankful if they can get their child to eat anything healthy at all. If you have to start cutting foods out of the diet because they appear to cause an allergic reaction or worsen asthma symptoms, then mealtimes can become particularly problematic.

Keep the following in mind.

- You should not be cutting foods out of your child's diet without being sure that they are contributing to your child's asthma. This requires the help of a dietitian or nutritional therapist, who will put your child on a monitored elimination diet (*see* chapter 2) and draw up a nutritious diet plan once an intolerance is established.

- Although your child may have a reaction to a certain food or foods, this may not mean they must be completely forbidden; an occasional treat may not cause an attack or worsening of symptoms, depending on the severity of the intolerance. But again this is something a dietitian or nutritional therapist will be able to help you work out.
- Using all the foods she can eat without problems, aim for as varied a diet as possible and keep putting previously spurned foods on her plate, even if she does not eat them and maintains that she does not like them. One day she might!
- Try to make the food attractive to your child: cut it into shapes (pastry cutters and plastic moulds are invaluable here), arrange it like a picture on the plate (a face, a sun, and so on). If it is fun to eat, she may just eat it.
- Do not become disheartened if she will not eat at mealtimes. It is difficult if you have spent time preparing a meal to find it is all wasted, but keep saying to yourself that it will not last for ever.
- Give vitamin drops (under three years) or children's vitamin pills as a safety net if you are worried that she is missing out on nutrients.
- Lastly, do not worry. Toddlers continue to thrive despite a somewhat haphazard diet – and have bags of energy, too.

Sleeping problems

Asthma symptoms can often be worse at night; experts are not sure why this is so, although it could be due to changes in hormones which occur at night or simply because there are more house-dust mites in bedding, triggering the symptoms. Whatever the causes, many anxious parents have spent nights by the bedside of a child who simply cannot sleep due to coughing and wheezing, or – once the child is asleep – sitting and listening to her breathe, wary that an attack could develop. It is not an easy situation for any parent to deal with and it can leave both you and your child screaming for one good night's sleep. There are some steps you can take, however.

- Follow the advice outlined in chapter 2 to lower the number of house-dust mites in the bedroom.
- Keep the air well-circulated, open a small window if possible (ie if it is not too cold or your child is not suffering from pollen exposure).
- Do not let your child get too hot.
- If mucus seems to be sitting on her chest, bolster up her pillows so that it has a chance to disperse; with babies, place a pillow under the cot mattress.
- If she is congested, place a saucer of water on a radiator with a few drops of decongestant essential oil in it (rosemary or eucalyptus).
- Things can seem worse in the dark, so invest in a night light for her room.
- If your child seems better when you are in the room, stay with her until she falls asleep. Make yourself comfortable while you wait, even if it means setting up a cot bed or sofa bed in the room ready for broken nights.
- Once she is asleep, go back to your room so that she does not expect you always to be with her. Be honest with her, however, about how long you are willing to stay in her room; explain that you will return to your own bed once she is asleep. This way, she will not wake up and panic because you are not there.
- Try to keep your own worries about her night asthma in perspective. It is easy in the wee small hours to dwell on the more negative possibilities but many children wheeze at night and asthmatic wheezers are better off than those whose symptoms stop them from sleeping altogether. To get a sense of perspective, try talking to your doctor, asthma nurse or complementary practitioner.
- A complementary therapist should also be able to help your child get a better night's sleep. Talk to her about the problem so

that she can tailor the treatment towards improving night symptoms.
- Finally, if things are really bad, you can get long-lasting medication from your doctor which will help your child get through the night.

Starting playgroup or nursery

Unless your child has been at a nursery or with a childminder from a younger age, you may start her at a playgroup or nursery at around three years old, and this will be the first time she will spend stretches of time away from you. Since she will probably only spend part of the day away, administering medication is not usually a problem at this stage, although she will need to keep her reliever with her; if your child attends full time, then refer to the next section for advice about schooling and medication.

You may find at this stage that she picks up more colds and other viruses, simply because she is mixing with more children. This may be a particular problem if she has no older brothers and sisters, who will have brought home their own infections and built up her resistance already. If colds bring on asthma, you might consider an anti-flu vaccination, although these are not recommended for the very young. A complementary therapist will also be able to build up her immunity so that she has more resistance to infection; a homeopath, for example, can offer remedies which protect in a similar but gentler way to an anti-flu vaccination. Beyond this, keep an eye on her asthma symptoms should a cold develop and be ready to increase her medication to ward off an attack.

Children under five should be encouraged to do all the things other toddlers and young children do: running about, climbing, jumping on the bed, riding a bike, chasing ducks, making friends and generally letting off steam. Get her mixing with other children at a playgroup, toddler club or nursery; build regular trips to the playpark into your day; join clubs – musical, mini-gymnastics, book reading – to keep her interested and stop her dwelling on symptoms. Join a Splash club or take your pre-schooler to the swimming pool every week – swimming is good for children with asthma, building up their lungs and helping with breathing as well as providing plenty of exercise splashing around.

Child-care checks

If your child goes to a nursery or childminder, you will need to check that:

- they can cope with an asthmatic child
- they know what to do in the event of an attack, or are willing to learn
- they are willing to give medication if necessary
- the environment does not contain potential allergens; this is particularly important when choosing a childminder, as your child will be in her home and she must be willing to make changes if she takes on your child

THE MIDDLE YEARS: FROM 5 TO 12

There are two major developments which occur in a child's life during these middle years. The first is starting school and the second puberty, and both can have a bearing on your child's life with asthma.

Starting school

Asthma is not a rarity in the classroom, particularly at the primary (first) school stage, when asthma is more prevalent. It is estimated that, in the UK, about 4 children in every class of 30 has asthma. It is also the most common reason for children needing to take medication at school. What is surprising for so common a condition is that so few schools have a policy on managing asthma and teachers themselves have so little knowledge of the condition. Surveys show that they generally have little awareness of what medication is used in asthma and how it can help in an attack, and some do not even know that asthma can be fatal. Many also cling to the outdated idea that asthma is psychosomatic.

A 1994 British conference, 'Asthma in the Classroom', identified a number of problems schools had with children with asthma. A major one was that many teachers and even school nurses were untrained in asthma and therefore vulnerable when an attack occurred. There were also problems about who should hold onto the inhaler and when a child would be allowed to use it, as well as a lack of understanding about how a child feels about having asthma and taking medication at school. The problems were not all with the school, however; parents, too, let the side down by not giving clear instructions about medication, not supplying the school with a reliever inhaler, or forgetting to give their child the inhaler to take to school.

Case Study
'I find schools the most difficult thing to cope with,' admits Lorraine, mother of five-year-old Darren. 'They really don't seem to know what they are doing and I have to write down instructions two or three times. We've also had problems with his medication. He was taking syrup when he started school, but the school wasn't prepared to give it to him – they wanted me to go in and do it. It just wasn't possible for me to go in two or three times a day in that way. So he changed to an inhaler, which he takes morning and evening, plus his reliever if he needs it – which goes to school with him.'

Because a positive policy towards children with asthma is so patchy and unregulated within the school system, parents need to do their own homework before deciding on a school for their child. When the time comes to choose a school, contact those in your area and ask:

• Do they have a policy on asthma? The policy should include an acknowledgement of the seriousness of the condition and a commitment to making the school environment favourable to children with it, including helping non-asthmatic children to understand it. It should also offer guidelines on what to do in the event of an asthma attack, and it should recognize the importance of a child having immediate access to her inhaler, preferably leaving it with the child herself when she is old enough to manage her own medication (around age seven).

- Have the staff – which includes teachers, the school secretary and the school nurse – had any training in dealing with asthma? An understanding of what causes asthma, how medication works and what to do in the event of an attack can greatly increase their confidence in having an asthmatic child in their class or school.

Check the school environment, too, for possible irritants, such as pets in the classroom, cigarette smoke from a nearby staffroom, vapours from the science laboratory, or mould spores if there is a problem with damp.

Do not be afraid to discuss your child's asthma at any preliminary meetings with both the head teacher and the class teacher, particularly if the school does not have a policy on asthma and the staff have no training in helping asthmatic children. Their responses will help you make a decision. If the school has an asthma policy, it will indicate whether it has any real meaning.

Being clear about asthma

If your child's school does not appear to have a very progressive policy on asthma and the teachers themselves show little knowledge on the subject, then it is down to you to fill the gap.

- Provide literature on asthma for the teacher to read, particularly anything which will dispel the myths which surround medication. Too many teachers still cling to the idea that asthma medications are dangerous. It needs to be made clear that an asthmatic child cannot overdose on asthma inhalers and there is no danger if friends have a puff – in fact, it can help take the mystery out of asthma for children who have not come across it at close quarters. You will find organizations which can provide this type of information under 'Useful addresses' at the end of the book.

- Give written guidelines to the school about your child's medication; it can be an annotated management plan, which will help the teacher recognize the symptoms of asthma and provide her with steps to take should an attack develop. Make sure the details are kept up to date.
- Be very clear about the need for medication to be accessible, whether it is held by the class teacher for younger children or by the child herself later on. Indicate times when extra medication may be necessary, for example before games, in winter when coming from cold air to warm, during the pollen season, and so on.

Any school or teacher that is committed to the welfare of pupils will be interested to learn more about asthma and want to help an asthmatic child; if you meet with opposition to a fair concern about your child's welfare, it may be wise to consider another school.

Your child's early experiences of school are important in developing her perceptions of herself and her asthma. Bad experiences at this age can dent her confidence and make her feel that she is not normal. Having to constantly ask the teacher for her inhaler or report to the school nurse's office at regular intervals for medication is one example of this; another is being prevented from joining in with games or school trips because of asthma. Perhaps the worst attitude children can encounter is being made to feel that they are putting on symptoms and should 'pull themselves together'. Asthma is a very real condition and needs sensitive handling on the part of the teachers.

Case Study

'Paul was perfectly all right at primary school but when he went to junior school a gang started bullying him about his asthma,' says his mother Laura. 'It wasn't anything physical, just name-calling and jibing, but it upset him terribly. He didn't want me to go up to the school but in the end I made an appointment to see his class teacher. She was totally unsympathetic, saying he would have to toughen up and even hinting that he 'put on' some of the symptoms. I was furious and had no hesitation in going to the head teacher. He was brilliant, talked to the boys involved, got an asthma nurse from a local clinic to give a talk and generally created a better climate for Paul at school. It's taught me that you have to be a bit pushy sometimes!'

It is well worth investing effort at this end of the schooling spectrum to send a confident teenager on to high school, one who knows she can control her asthma and that it does not stop her from doing anything her friends are doing.

Holidays

As children get older, families tend to become more adventurous when it comes to holidays. If your child has asthma, going on holiday, particularly abroad, is often a worry: what if the excitement, the strange environment, changes in diet, increased exercise, climatic and atmospheric conditions, even the stress of not being at home, leads to an attack? But there is no reason why this should happen as long as the asthma is under control before you go (that is, there are no signs of an imminent attack) and you take a few simple precautions.

- Think about what triggers your child's asthma before deciding on a destination and time of year to go. Skiing may be out if your child reacts badly to cold air; a walking or biking holiday is not advisable during the pollen season, if pollens are a particular problem; high-altitude holidays, where the air is thinner, are probably best avoided if your child's asthma is easily aggravated by air changes. Activity holidays may also present a problem if asthma is triggered by exercise. Scuba diving in particular is not usually recommended for asthmatics, because it places pressure on the lungs; consult your doctor before allowing your child to try it.
- Get your child checked over before you go by your complementary therapist, to get her body in fighting-fit form to challenge any environmental or other triggers.

- Take a good supply of her medication with you – preventers, relievers and spacer if required, as well as her peak flow meter. You might also consider taking a back-up prescription of steroid tablets in case of an emergency but discuss this with your doctor first. Keep to her normal medication and monitoring regime as much as possible. In addition, ask your doctor to fill in an asthma card, giving details of your child's medication; asthma cards are available from doctors or from asthma organizations.

- Check with your doctor or the embassy of the country you are visiting that there are no problems getting through customs with your child's medication. The most common holiday destinations should not be a problem; it is only if you are going somewhere more exotic that you may need to double-check. Getting a note from your doctor that the drugs are for personal use may be recommended. Inhalers can be carried on planes, despite what is said about pressurized containers; carry them with you in your hand luggage so that they do not get too cold.

- Make sure you have adequate holiday medical insurance to cover emergency hospital treatment. Check that the policy covers asthma.

- When you get to your destination, find out where to go for medical help, for example how to contact the hotel doctor or where the nearest hospital is.

- If asthma symptoms start, do not panic! Asthma is a global phenomenon and doctors worldwide are experienced in its treatment; in many countries, the drugs used are the same, even though they may go under different brand names. If there are language difficulties and no translator is available, use your child's asthma card to provide details of current medication and dosage, or write down what medication your child takes so that the dosage is clear to the doctor.

- Lastly, but most important, *try to relax*. It is what you go on holiday for, after all, and seeing you constantly on tender-hooks will not help your child to relax and enjoy herself, either!

■ Parties and socializing

Once children go to school, they will be going out of the house more socially as well as during the school day. And as they grow older they will not relish you going with them. This socializing inevitably means that they will be exposed to a range of triggers – pets, foods, house-dust mites and so on – which may cause an attack. You do not want to stop your child from going out and spreading her wings, so take steps to minimize the chances of an attack.

- Make sure your child is aware of what triggers her asthma so that she can avoid it. You can even teach her what to say in situations where she has to refuse something – for example, 'I'm sorry, but I can't go into the garden/eat chocolate/hold the kittens, because it affects my asthma.'
- If she becomes overexcited before going out and this stress brings on asthma, do some relaxing exercises to calm her down (*see* chapter 3).
- If necessary she could take a puff of medication before going into a trigger-heavy environment, for example, a house with pets or where she may be involved in energetic play.
- Ask your complementary therapist if there are any remedies she can recommend for quick back-up help, for example flower remedies to regulate overexcitement, an acupressure technique or a homeopathic remedy.

■ Sports and exercise

Keeping active is important if you have asthma. Gone are the days when children were thought to be too feeble to join in; now we know that playing sports and getting plenty of exercise help to build up children's stamina, muscles and lung power so that they become more resistant to asthma symptoms, as well as helping to boost their growth rate.

Case Study

'I tend to get asthma if I run around a lot, as well as in the cold,' says 11-year-old Nichola. 'But I do karate and have done it for quite a long time now, and that actually helps. It builds up your lungs and you do breathing exercises.'

Swimming is particularly good as it builds up the lungs and helps breathing.

For many people with asthma, exercise can bring on symptoms (exercise-induced asthma), but this is no bar to playing sports, as long as your child gets into the habit of preparing for it by taking extra medication beforehand and keeping her asthma under good control generally by following the many suggestions outlined in this book. It also helps to have a warm-up – a few 30-second sprints spaced over five to ten minutes – before starting exercise.

Going into puberty

The good news about puberty – that stage when a child undergoes the physical and emotional changes of emerging adulthood – is that many children, particularly boys, lose their asthma. For many others, the symptoms die down and become much easier to manage, in some cases allowing a child to drop preventers altogether, only using her reliever when needed.

On the other hand, puberty can be delayed in children with asthma, which means they may lag behind their classmates in terms of stature and body changes. We do not know why this occurs, although both uncontrolled asthma and prolonged use of high-dose steroids can affect growth. However, teenagers with asthma catch up later on, with a longer period of growth, and reach their projected height by the time they are in their early twenties.

Menstruation may affect girls' asthma, with symptoms getting worse just before and during a period. Doctors believe that this may be linked to hormonal changes around menstruation, specifically to drops in the female hormone oestrogen. Once your daughter's periods have settled into a cycle, it may be worth keeping a diary of peak flow readings and asthma symptoms along with menstruation dates. You will then see if there is a link between menstrual cycle and asthma symptoms and can talk to your doctor about increasing medication around that time. Complementary therapies designed to help regulate the hormonal cycle, like homeopathy, acupuncture and nutritional therapy, can also help.

Children with asthma are, of course, the same as other children when it comes to the emotional upheavals of puberty, but asthma can cause some additional turmoils. Resistance to taking medication may set in, even though your child knows it keeps her asthma at bay. She may feel her inhaler marks her out as different at a time when the need to fit in is paramount; an inhaler does not tend to give a teenager much 'street cred'. It is also a time of testing the rules that you have laid down, trying to knock down the fences and become independent. This may mean that she uses her medication as a way of getting to you and testing your reactions. Although it may be difficult, you need to be particularly understanding and supportive at this time, while quietly monitoring your child's progress. Gentle reminders of the advantages of taking medication regularly may be all you need, as most children are well aware of the miseries of an asthma attack. Remind her, for example, that making sure her asthma is well controlled with preventive medication means never having to use her reliever when she is out with friends.

Keeping a check on medication

As your child gets older, she will want to take responsibility for her own health and treatment. When you hand medication over to her depends on her personality; you have to judge when she is mature enough to manage it on her own without misuse (forgetting to take it, overusing her reliever, not keeping her reliever with her, and so on) and to spot any signs that her asthma is not as well controlled as it should be. Around seven years old seems to be the average for taking this step, but a more mature child may be able to do it at a younger age. However, even if she seems to be handling the responsibility well, it pays to keep a discreet eye out for problems. Look out for:

- how much medication is being used up – you will soon become adept at knowing how long it takes before canisters need replacing and will register if this is not happening as often as or more often than it should
- signs that your child is using her reliever more than usual – it means her symptoms are not being kept under control by preventers.
- erratic PEF readings (lower in the morning, varying by more than 15 per cent, below 80 per cent of her best reading).

THE TEENAGE YEARS: FROM 13 TO 18

Now is the time when children turn into adults and start taking over the reins of their life. As I have said, many teenagers are lucky enough to find that the symptoms of asthma disappear or become milder. For others, it means continuing with the routine that they have got used to over the years, avoiding triggers and knowing when asthma symptoms need a little extra control. Some children develop asthma for the first time now, which means getting into a routine and making additional changes to their life. Most children who develop asthma at this stage quickly take over responsibility for their health care and adapt. What the majority of teenagers with asthma have in common, whether they have had the condition some time or it has just developed, is a steely determination that it is not going to stop them doing what they want to do in life. And really – unless it is severe – it will not do so.

Sports and exercise

It is at this stage that children become more serious about sports. No sport is banned because of asthma, except those which involve the use of pressurized air like scuba diving. Activities associated with high altitudes, like mountaineering and in some cases skiing, may cause problems, because the air is thinner at altitude, but there is no reason why your child cannot try them. It really depends on her asthma, the triggers which bring it on and how severe the symptoms are. With asthma, it is always down to the individual and you and your child are the best people to know what her body can take, and you can always discuss it with your doctor if you are unsure.

School trips
Older children usually go on more – and longer – organized outings, whether it is a skiing holiday or a geography field trip. This may pose more of a problem than a one-day trip because it places your child in a different environment, with a variety of new triggers, and adds stress, excitement and even unaccustomed exercise. But having asthma should not mean she always has to miss out, unless it is a trip which would obviously put her in the path of triggers – for example, a field trip at the height of the pollen season. Beyond this, it just means being prepared.

- Make sure your child's asthma is well controlled before she goes away. Take regular peak flow measurements in the month beforehand and take steps quickly if she is not performing as well as normal. Complementary therapies can help get her into peak condition if she has been seeing a therapist regularly up to this point.
- Make sure she takes her medication with her, that she has enough for the time she is going to be away, and that she keeps her usual medication routine, even though she is away from home. She should not let being around her classmates put her off. If she is in a dormitory and feels shy about using her puffer in front of others, she should ask whoever is in charge if there is somewhere private she can go to take her regular dose of preventer.
- Let whoever is in charge know she has asthma, where she keeps her medication and what to do in an emergency. An asthma card can be helpful as a visual reminder to the teacher if an asthma attack occurs.
- She should take her reliever medication with her wherever she goes just in case. In a new environment, she may find she needs it even though the asthma seems to be well controlled.
- Encourage her to relax, enjoy herself and not worry about having an asthma attack.

Case Study

'Lee uses his reliever before and after sport,' says Trudie of her sports-mad 14-year-old football champion. 'He doesn't have any problems then.' There are many professional sportsmen and women who have asthma, control it well and win medals in their chosen field.

Stress

The teenage years mark an increase in the level of stress and tension young people experience, principally from pressure to achieve academically or in sports, to keep up with their friends socially or to pass examinations. Your child's relationship with you may also become more stressful, as she starts to be more independent and friction develops between what she wants to do and what you would like her to do. There is also stress in establishing her first close relationships outside the family, having a boyfriend, making the first moves, even telling him about her asthma. And the physical changes of adolescence can also be a cause of stress.

There is no doubt that stress can trigger asthma for some people and it is bound to happen that, as soon as there is something important coming up (an examination, a big sports event, a first date), the tension will cause your child to feel stressed and asthma symptoms will start appearing. So you need to know how to cut down on stress where possible, and control it when it occurs. The stress management techniques outlined in chapter 3 will help with this and give you ideas for a plan of action. You can also draw on complementary therapies which have a track record in cutting down on stress, like yoga, massage, aromatherapy, reflexology or acupuncture (*see* chapter 5).

Teenage stress points

- examinations
- arguments with parents
- homework
- spots
- sports competitions
- dating
- driving lessons
- sex
- money worries

Choosing a career

Probably the biggest question during these years is: What am I going to do with my life? In answering it, your child may have to take her asthma into consideration although, again, it depends on her and her asthma. She should bear her triggers in mind when fixing on a career. For example, a job outdoors (gardener, building work, etc) is not advisable if her asthma is triggered by pollens, particularly if it is a broad spectrum of pollens which may put her out of service for most of the summer and autumn. Working with animals may pose a problem for anyone whose asthma is triggered by animal dander. Since air quality is so vital to asthma control, dusty, fume-filled or smoky environments are also risky; wood dust, adhesives like those found in spray paints, lacquers and polyurethanes, and foods like flour and grains have been found to pose particular problems. The emergency services (police, fire and ambulance) are also wary about employing someone who currently has asthma, although it may be worth your child's while applying if she had asthma as a child but it has now cleared up; likewise with the armed forces.

Missed schooling

Days or even weeks out from school are not crucial for younger children, but as they get older and school work translates into grades and examinations, keeping up takes on greater significance. Children with asthma do tend to take more time off school: one study found that 58 per cent of asthmatic children have at least some days off school over a 12-month period with 12 per cent losing more than 30 days. Unfortunately, catching up takes a lot of hard work.

- Do not allow your child to take time off unnecessarily; it is a temptation for anyone to feign illness and take a few days off now and again, but it is simply more lost time.
- Ask teachers for work she can do at home. In this way, she will stay in touch with what is happening in the classroom, not get too far behind, and show the teachers that she is committed to her schoolwork. This will ideally motivate them to help her, even if it means putting in a little extra time.

- If she has work to do while at home, make sure she does it. It is easy for a child to turn into a couch potato, glued to the TV or a computer screen, but she must learn to be strong with herself. If she uses the time constructively she will have less to do when she gets back to school.
- Encourage her to keep in touch, and ask friends to come around after school to go through what has been covered in the class. Just because she has an asthma attack does not mean she has to go into isolation!
- Think positive and try not to become depressed about the situation. Work at getting the asthma under control and then let your child go back to her schoolwork with a new sense of energy, putting the attack behind her and getting on with her life.

Social life

Asthma need not put a damper on your child's social life as she grows older, although smoky environments like those in a pub or club are likely to cause problems. If she is going to spend time in a smoky atmosphere and it affects her asthma, she should take extra medication beforehand, keep her reliever with her and sit where she is not surrounded by smokers, if possible by an entrance so that fresh air is coming in. Then she should try to balance the effects of the smoke by getting as much fresh air into her lungs the day after. If she finds she really cannot put up with the smokiness, she may have to avoid these places or just stay a short time; in this case, she should evolve a social life which does not revolve around pubs and clubs, for example sports activities, computer clubs, drama, music and so on.

It goes without saying that anyone with asthma should not smoke, and your child may also find that she has to be careful with alcohol. Some people with asthma find that alcohol can bring on symptoms.

Sex

Many young adults with asthma worry that the condition will have an effect on their sex life, but it is only occasionally a problem. In a few cases, the exertions of sex may cause breathlessness and an increase in symptoms particularly if the asthma is exercise-induced. Symptoms can also occur because of house-dust mites in the bedding, in which case you or your child will need to take the practical steps outlined in chapter 2 to cut down on the house-dust mite population. Beyond this, a worsening of asthma during sex could be psychosomatic: if your child is worried that asthma will interfere with intercourse and feels stressed because of it, then symptoms are likely to develop. Learning to relax and get her worries into perspective will help here.

Moving away from home

At around 18, many teenagers strike out on their own for the first time, whether going to university or taking a job away from home. This is a big step; suddenly they are managing their own money, cooking for themselves, making a host of everyday decisions which were previously taken care of by their parents, even something as simple as getting themselves up in time for work or classes is a challenge for a lot of teenagers.

This is a difficult time for you as well. You will no longer be able to keep a friendly eye on your child and will quite naturally be worried about her – asthma will be only one of your concerns.

Case Study
'My mum was driving me mad,' says 24-year-old Maddie, who left home for university at the age of 18. 'She phoned me every evening. At first, it was comforting to hear her voice because I did feel a bit lost and lonely. But after a month, it was getting a bit much, particularly since it was obvious she wasn't phoning about me, she was phoning about my asthma. I felt fine, I had no asthma symptoms, I was busy settling in, but every time we spoke, Mum would ram my asthma at me: 'How is your asthma? You don't have a cold, do you? Do you have enough medication? I felt like she was almost wishing there was something wrong with me, so I'd have to come home.' Maddie let the situation continue for a few more weeks before a visit

home, when, she says, 'I had it out with her. I guess it had been bubbling inside me that she didn't really trust me. We had an argument which ended with my mum breaking down in tears. Finally, she admitted that she couldn't stop thinking about my asthma, reliving the attacks I had as a child, dreaming up nightmare scenarios of me having an asthma attack with no one there to help me. I suddenly saw my leaving home from her point of view.'

For asthmatic teenagers, moving away from home means really taking responsibility for their lives and health. You will not be there to check that your child has a good supply of medication, or to nag her into keeping an eye on her asthma. She will have a new routine, new friends to explain her asthma to. But you must give her her independence. Growing up and knowing that she is on top of the asthma will help her to grow in self-confidence.

There are people with asthma in all walks of life, from actors, politicians and sportsmen and women to doctors, journalists and teachers, and for the most part one would not know that they had asthma. Asthma is as much about attitude of mind as it is anything else. Once your child knows that asthma is not going to get in her way, life takes off.

Further Reading

Anxiety, Phobias and Panic Attacks by Elaine Sheehan (Element, 1996)

Asthma in the Classroom: A report prepared by the Schools Health Education Unit, University of Exeter (National Asthma Training Centre, 1994)

Asthma: Who Cares? In the Home: A Manual to Help Parents Whose Children Have Asthma (National Asthma Training Centre, 1995)

Creating Kids Who Can by Jean Robb and Hilary Letts (Hodder & Stoughton, 1995)

The Elimination Diet Cookbook by Jill Carter and Alison Edwards (Element, 1997)

Overcoming Anxiety by Helen Kennerley (Robinson, 1997)

'Symptom, Perception and Evaluation in Childhood Asthma. Nursing Research' by H. Lorrie Voos and Ann McMullen, in *Paediatric Nursing,* 22, 4, p 285 (8)

Thorax: The British Guidelines on Asthma Management, 1995 Review and Position Statement (BMJ Publishing Group, 1995)

Which? Guide to Complementary Medicine by Barbara Rowlands (Which? Books, 1997).

What Doctors Don't Tell You by Lynne McTaggart (Thorsons, 1996)

Useful Addresses

International

International Federation of Reflexologists
78 Edridge Rd
Croydon
Surrey CR0 1EF
Tel: 0181 667 9458

La Lèche League International
PO Box 1209
Franklin Park
IL 60131-8209

Australia

Allergy Association of Australia
PO Box 214
North Beach
WA 6020

Australian Natural Therapists Association
7 Highview Grove
Burwood East
VIC 3151

Australian Traditional Medicine Society
120 Blaxland Rd,
Ryde,
NSW 2112

Marriage and Family Counselling Service
2262 Pitt Street
Sydney
NSW 2000

Nursing Mothers Association of Australia
16 Dinsdale Place
Hamersley
WA 6022

Canada

AIA Allergy Information Association
3 Powburn Place
Weston
Ontario

Canadian Association for Marriage and Family Therapy
271 Russell Hill Road
Toronto
Ontario
M4V 2T5

Canadian Holistic Medical Association
42 Redpath Ave
Toronto
Ontario
M4S 2J6

Secrétariat Général de la Léche League
CF P 874
Ville St Laurent
Québec
H4L 4W3

Canadian Institute of Stress
1235 Bay St
Toronto
Ontario
M5R 3K4

United Kingdom

Action Against Allergy
43 The Downs
London
SW20 8HG
Information and leaflets on allergic conditions.

Aromatherapy Organisations Council
3 Latymer Close
Braybrooke
Market Harborough
Leics
LE16 8LN
Tel: 01858 434242

British Acupuncture Council
Park House
206/208 Latimer Rd
London
W10 6RE
Tel: 0181 964 0222

British Association for Autogenic Training and Therapy
Heath Cottage
Pitch Hill
Ewhurst nr Cranleigh
Surrey
GU6 7NP

British Association for Counselling
37a Sheep St
Rugby
Warks
CV21 3BX
Tel: 01788 578328

British Massage Therapy Council
Greenbank House
65a Adelphi St
Preston
PR1 7BH
Tel: 01772 881063

British Wheel of Yoga
1 Hamilton Place
Boston Rd
Sleaford
Lincs
NG34 7ES
Tel: 01529 306851

General Council and Register of Consultant Herbalists
18 Sussex Square
Brighton
East Sussex
BN2 5AA
Tel: 01243 267126

General Council and Register of Naturopaths
Goswell House
2 Goswell Rd
Street
Somerset
BA16 0JG
Tel: 01458 840072

Institute for Complementary Medicine
PO Box 194
London
SE14 1QZ
Tel: 0171 237 5165

La Lèche League
BM 3424
London
WC1V 6XX
Tel: 0171 242 1278
Support for breastfeeding mothers.

National Asthma Campaign
Providence House
Providence Place
London
N1 0NT
Asthma helpline: 0345 010203

Provides leaflets and literature; runs local support groups, holiday for children
and the Junior Asthma Club.

National Asthma Training Centre
Winton House
Church Street
Stratford-upon-Avon
Warwickshire
CV37 6HB
Provides information for health professionals and schools; publishes *Asthma Who Cares? In the Home*, a guide for parents who have children with asthma.

National Childbirth Trust
Alexandra House
Oldham Terrace
London
W3 6NH
Tel: 0181 992 8637
Support for pregnant women, breastfeeding mothers and those with young children.

National Council of Psychotherapists and Hypnotherapists
46 Oxhey Rd
Oxhey
Watford
Herts
WD1 4QQ

National Eczema Society
163 Eversholt Street
London
NW1 1BU
Information and support for children with eczema.

Osteopathic Information Service
PO Box 2074
Reading
Berks
RG1 4YR
Tel: 01491 875255

Quitline
102 Gloucester Place
London
W1H 3DA
Tel: 0800 002200
For support and advice on quitting smoking.

RELATE
Herbert Gray College
Little Church Street
Rugby
Warwickshire
CV21 3AP
For marital, relationship and family problems.

Society for the Promotion of Nutritional Therapy
PO Box 47
Heathfield
East Sussex
TN21 8ZX
Tel: 01435 867007

Society of Homoeopaths
2 Artizan Rd
Northampton
NN1 4HU
Tel: 01604 21400

Society of Teachers of the Alexander Technique
20 London House
266 Fulham Rd
London
SW10 9EL
Tel: 0171 351 0828

Yoga Therapy Centre
Royal London Homeopathic Hospital
60 Great Ormond St
London
WC1N 3HR
Tel: 0171 833 7267

United States

Asthma and Allergy Foundation of America
1717 Massachusetts Avenue
Suite 305
Washington DC 20036

American Lung Association
1740 The Broadway
New York
NY10019 4374

National Anxiety Foundation
3135 Custer Drive
Lexington
Kentucky 40517

La Leche League International
PO Box 1209
Franklin Park
IL 60131-8209

Index

acaricide 28
acupuncture 22, 44, 71, 72, 76–7,
    84, 102, 105
  laser 77
  ultrasound 77
acupressure 77, 100
adenoids 16
adhesives 13, 106
adrenal glands 64, 65
adrenal suppression 64, 65, 66
air 1, 2, 4, 6, 16, 25, 27, 28, 31, 42,
    98, 103, 107
  circulation 8, 25, 26, 92
  cold viii, 1, 6, 9, 13, 15, 97, 98
  filters 27, 28
  pollution 1, 8, 9, 11, 71
  quality 9, 106
  travel 99
  warm 6, 9
airways 1, 2, 3, 14, 15, 16, 18, 30,
    55, 56, 82, 84, 86
alcohol 107
Alexander technique 40, 75,
    77–78
allergens 1, 3, 4, 5, 6, 9, 13, 20,
    21, 25, 28, 34, 35, 71, 78, 82,
    83, 94

allergies 11, 13, 29, 32, 78
allergy clinics 36, 56, 60
altitudes 98, 103
anaphylactic shock 11
animal 21, 31
  dander 2, 4, 13, 20, 28, 29, 106
  fats 32
antibiotics 13, 16
antibodies 2, 32, 89
anti-inflammatories 55, 56
anxiety 36–45, 49, 53, 66, 72
Archives of Diseases in
    Childhood 9
Armed forces 106
aromatherapy 44, 82, 105
asthma
  acute 13, 63, 80
  allergic 1, 13, 18, 21
  attacks vii, viii, ix, 3, 13, 15, 17,
    18, 19, 28, 38, 39, 42, 43, 45,
    50, 56, 60, 65, 66, 67–8, 73,
    81, 84, 86, 87, 91, 93, 94, 95,
    96, 97, 98, 100, 104
  brittle 19, 61
  cards 64, 99, 104
  chronic 5, 13, 19
  clinic 60, 73

exercise-induced 5–6, 48,
    101, 108
extrinsic 13
intrinsic 13
mild 1, 5, 15, 17, 19, 65, 72
moderate 19, 48, 65
night-time 14, 15, 57, 91–3
nurse 17, 18, 74, 92
occupational 13
rates viii
severe 1, 15, 17, 19, 55, 56, 57,
    63, 65, 67, 73
viral 13, 18
atopic conditions ix, 10, 16
Autogenic training 75, 78

beclomethasone 56
bedding 4, 24, 26, 27, 91, 108
beds 24, 26, 29, 92
beta2-agonists 57, 66
Bio-resonance therapy 78
breastfeeding 32, 89, 90
breathing 58, 66, 72, 77, 94, 101
    difficulties ix, 14, 16, 39, 42, 43,
        47, 67, 69
    exercises 41, 42, 43, 85
    overbreathing 42, 43, 86–7
    shallow 42, 43, 85
breathlessness 1, 13, 14, 15,
    19, 108
British Allergy Foundation 27
British Medical Journal 8, 29
bronchiolitis 15
bronchitis 16
bronchoconstriction 1
bronchodilators 55, 56–7, 64
    long-acting 56
    short-acting 57
bronchospasm 1

bruising 65, 66
budesonide 56
bunk beds 24
Buteyko method 75, 86–7

carbon dioxide 2, 42, 43, 86
careers 13, 88, 106
carpeting 4, 23, 24, 26
cataracts 66
Center for Disease Control and
    Prevention 11
central heating 8–9, 25
challenge testing 35
chemicals 8, 10, 11, 12, 25, 83
chest
    pain 14, 42
    tightness 6, 14, 19, 42
childminders 93, 94
chimneys 8, 25
clothing 4, 24, 25, 31, 41
cockroaches 7
colds, see infections
communication 51
complementary therapists ix, 15,
    19, 20, 43–4, 45, 52, 65, 66,
    71–87, 88, 92, 93, 98, 100,
    102, 104, 105
    choosing 74–5
    doctor's attitudes 71, 73
    qualifications 74
    regulatory bodies 74
compost heaps 30
confidence 48, 49, 50, 96, 97,
    98, 109
Consumers' Association 27, 71
corticosteroids 19, 56, 63, 66,
    68, 99
    side effects 32, 64–6
cortisone 64

coughing viii, 1, 6, 13, 14, 15, 16, 19, 43, 66, 67, 91
counselling 44, 53
cromolyn sodium, *see* sodium cromoglycate
croup 16
curtains 23, 24, 26
Cushing's syndrome 66
customs 99
cystic fibrosis 16

dairy products 33, 34, 35, 36, 90
damp 8, 25, 31, 96
dander, *see* animal dander
dating 105
depression 7, 39, 43, 107
diabetes 64, 66
diagnosis viii, 13–17, 20, 76, 88
diet ix, 11, 31–3, 45, 65, 76, 83, 98
    babies 89–90
    elimination diet 21, 35, 36, 83, 91
    for toddlers 33, 90–1
    plans 36, 84
dietitian 10, 21, 33, 35, 36, 90, 91
dizziness 42
driving 105
dust 8, 25, 26, 27, 28

eczema ix, 2, 11, 16, 32, 34
emergencies 15, 17, 18, 63, 67, 68–9, 104
emergency services
    calling 15, 17, 45, 68
    a career in 106
emotions 20, 38, 51, 72, 82, 84, 102
    as triggers 7, 72
    children 38, 46–8

teenagers 46–8
parents vii, 38, 49–51
environment 1, 8, 11, 13, 22, 44, 88, 94, 95, 96, 98, 100, 104
epilepsy 40
essential oils 28, 79, 82, 92
excitement 7, 98, 100, 104
exercise viii, 1, 5–6, 13, 14, 15, 45, 94, 97, 98, 100–1, 103–4

face masks 58, 61
family
    balance 51
    history 2, 16, 34, 50, 89
    therapy 53
fatalities ix, 46, 47, 50, 52
fatigue 11, 14, 65, 83
feelings *see* emotions
fireplaces 8, 25
flower remedies 82, 100
fluticasone 56
food
    additives 10, 11, 32, 33, 35, 83
    allergy 10–11, 13, 16, 21, 32, 33–6, 83, 89, 90, 100
    diary 21, 34, 35
    intolerance 10–11, 13, 20, 21, 33–6, 83, 84, 91
    withdrawal 35
formula milk 11, 32, 89, 90
furnishings 4, 8, 23, 24, 29

gardens 30–1
gas stoves 9, 25
genetic susceptibility viii, ix, 2, 55
glaucoma 64, 66
grass 5, 30, 31
growth 6, 31, 64, 65, 66, 100, 101
guilt vii, 50

hay fever ix, 2, 4–5, 16, 27, 29
headaches 64, 66, 83
heart rate 7, 64, 66
hedges 30
herbal medicine 75
    Chinese 76–7
    Western 79–80
herbs 75, 77, 79, 83
    dangers of 79
    over the counter 73
holidays 7, 98–9
home 8–9
    environment ix, 4, 23–8,
        88, 94
    moving away from 88, 108–9
homeopathy 44, 71, 75, 80–1, 83,
    93, 100, 102
homework 105, 106
hospital 17, 64, 68, 69–70, 99
house-dust mites 3, 4, 7, 9, 11, 13,
    15, 20, 23, 24, 26, 27, 28, 91,
    92, 100, 108
houses 8–9
    moving 9
hyperactivity 10, 66
hyperventilation 42–3
hypnotherapy 22, 40, 44, 75, 81–2
    hypnohealing 82
    self-hypnosis 81–2
hypoxia 62

immune system ix, 2, 8, 11, 12, 32,
    36, 65, 71, 83
immunity 9, 12, 64, 65, 66, 93
immunotherapy 56
infections 1, 3, 11, 12, 13, 15–16,
    18, 34, 65, 67, 71, 93
inflammation 1, 2, 56, 72, 82,
    83, 86

inhalers 32, 47, 56, 57, 58, 59, 61,
    62, 63, 66, 95, 96, 97, 99, 102
International Study of Asthma &
    Allergy in Children
    (ISAAC) viii
ionisers 27
ipratropium bromide 57

Journal of Epidemiology &
    Community Health 6

La Lèche League 89
laughter 7
lethargy 14, 34, 35, 42, 69
lungs vii, 1, 2, 16, 39, 62, 63, 76,
    85, 86, 94, 98, 101, 107

management plan 17–18, 43, 45,
    52, 67, 68, 97
massage therapy 44, 75, 76, 79,
    82, 105
mattresses 4, 15, 24, 26, 27, 92
MDI, *see* inhalers
medical herbalism, *see* herbal
    medicine
medication 5, 6, 14, 17, 19, 45, 47,
    49, 50, 57–64, 65, 72, 73, 75,
    79, 87, 88, 93, 94, 95, 96, 97,
    99, 100, 101, 102–3, 104,
    107, 109
meditation 44, 82, 86
menstruation 101, 102
meridians 76
minerals 31, 36–7, 73, 83
    calcium 32
    magnesium 37
moulds 5, 8, 30, 31, 96
moxibustion 77
mucus 1, 3, 14, 16, 56, 84, 92

muscle
  spasm 1, 56, 72, 84
  tremor 66
  wasting 66
  weakness 66

National Asthma Campaign 27, 30
National Asthma Training Centre 58
naturopathy 82–3
nausea 11, 66
nebulisers 61–2, 68, 69
nedocromil 56
nursery 93–4
nutritional
  deficiencies 31, 36, 83
  status 83
  therapy 21, 33, 35, 36, 83–4, 90, 91, 102
nuts 33, 36

osteopathy 71, 75, 83, 84
osteoporosis 32, 64, 66
over-anxiety 49–50
oxygen 1, 2, 7, 14, 42, 43, 68, 69, 86

pallor 69
panic 18, 43, 68, 81, 92
parties 100
peak flow 16–17, 57, 67, 68, 99, 102, 103, 104
peanuts 11, 36
pesticides 10, 33
pets 3, 4, 7, 9, 16, 20, 28–9, 31, 96, 100
pilates 40
plants 5, 25, 30–31

playgroup 7, 93–4
pollen 2, 3, 4–5, 6, 11, 13, 15, 16, 20, 21, 24, 25, 27, 29–31, 67, 92, 97, 98, 104, 106
polyunsaturated fatty acids 37
polyurethane 106
positive thinking 45–6, 47, 49, 52, 82
posture 39–40, 77, 78, 84
  postural therapies 40, 75, 85
prednisolone 56, 63, 66
preschoolers 88–94
preventers 19, 56, 63, 66, 99, 101, 103, 104
puberty 7, 94, 101–3
  delayed 101
puffer, see inhaler

qi 76

radiators 25
rashes 11, 83
reflexology 44, 75, 84–5, 105
relationships
  with boy/girl friend 7, 105
  with parents 54, 102, 105
relaxation 39, 40–2, 72, 75, 82, 83, 85, 86, 99, 100, 104, 108
  deep 78, 81
  programme 41–2
  tapes 40
relievers 19, 49, 55, 56, 61, 63, 64, 66, 67, 68, 93, 95, 99, 101, 102, 103, 104, 107
responsibility
  fear of 50–1
  taking 20, 47, 49, 51, 54, 61, 88, 102, 103, 109

rewards 60
rhinitis ix
routines 22, 52, 63, 103, 104

sadness 7, 39
salbutamol 57, 63
salmeterol 56
school 7, 46, 47, 48–9, 52, 64, 88,
    93, 100, 105
  examinations 7, 88, 105, 106
  missed 47, 106–7
  nurse 64, 95, 96, 97
  policy on asthma 94–6
  starting 49, 94–98
  trips 97, 104
scuba diving 98, 103
sealed covers 24, 26, 27
self-esteem 48–9
sex 105, 107–8
siblings 21, 51, 53, 54, 69, 93
side effects
  of medication 32, 57, 62,
    63, 64–6
  of vaccinations 11, 12
silent chest 69
skiing 98, 103, 104
skin
  prick testing 21
  thinning 64, 66
sleep 11, 91–93
smoking 5, 8, 15, 16, 22–3, 81,
    96, 107
socializing 22, 100, 107
sodium cromoglycate 56, 63, 66
spacers 58, 59, 68, 99
sports 57, 100–101, 103–104,
    105, 107
spray paints 13, 106
steroids, *see* corticosteroids

stress 6, 7, 11, 13, 38–45, 53, 72,
    77, 78, 81, 82, 83, 85, 98,
    100, 104, 105, 108
supplements 36–7, 73, 84
swimming 94, 101
symptom diary, *see* food diary
symptoms viii, ix, 1, 4, 5, 6, 7, 8,
    10, 13, 14, 15, 16, 17, 18, 19,
    20, 21, 23, 25, 27, 28, 31, 34,
    35, 36, 38, 39, 42, 43, 44, 45,
    47, 50, 52, 55, 56, 57, 60, 63,
    66, 67, 68, 69, 72, 73, 76,
    80, 81, 85, 86, 88, 90, 91, 93,
    97, 99, 101, 102, 103, 104,
    105, 108

t'ai chi 44, 76, 82
teachers 48, 49, 64, 94, 95, 96,
    97, 106
teenagers 18, 47, 75, 78, 88,
    98, 103–9
terbutaline 57, 63
theophylline 57, 66
thrush 11, 66
thunderstorms 6
tingling 42
tiredness, *see* Fatigue
toys 4, 15, 25, 26, 70
toxic overload 10, 83
Traditional Chinese medicine 44,
    76–7, 84
trembling 42, 64
triggers viii, ix, 1, 2–13, 14, 15,
    16, 19, 20, 21, 22, 26, 27, 29,
    31, 44, 67, 73, 98, 100, 103,
    104, 106

vaccinations 11–12, 16
  anti-influenza 93

vaccinations (*continued*)
  MMR 11
  DTP 11
  BCG 12
vacuum cleaners 27
vacuuming 24, 25, 26
vaporizers 28, 82
ventilation 8, 31
visualization 40–2, 43
vitamins 31, 36–7, 73, 83, 91
  antioxidants 32, 37
  betacarotene 32, 37
  B6 37
  C 32, 37
  E 32, 37
vomiting 11, 66

washing 24, 25, 26
water
  pollution 10
  retention 66
weaning 89–90
weather 6, 21, 98
weight 11, 65, 66
'What Doctors Don't Tell You' 11
wheat products 33, 34, 35, 36, 90
wheezing viii, 6, 13, 14, 15, 16, 19,
    43, 67, 69, 91, 92
whooping cough 12, 16
wood dust 12, 13, 106

yin and yang 75, 76
yoga 41, 44, 75, 85–6, 105